Praise for *The Good Karma Diet*

"Every one of Victori[...] [...]s people, animals, and the earth. [...]tion—it's eminently readable, highly in[...] [...] useful."

—Gene Stone, author of *The Secrets of People Who Never Get Sick*
and the #1 *New York Times* bestseller *Forks over Knives*

"*The Good Karma Diet* solves your food questions and diet challenges with a fun, practical, and remarkably simple approach. If you'd like to ramp up your motivation and accelerate your success, this refreshing and uplifting book will be the one to do it."

—Neal D. Barnard, MD, founder of Physicians Committee for Responsible Medicine
and author of the *New York Times* bestseller *21-Day Weight Loss Kickstart*

"Victoria Moran is an inspiration to all who know her, and *The Good Karma Diet* gets the formula right: combine food that's full of life, a heart that's full of love, and expect to experience joy, vitality, and beauty at every age."

—Mimi Kirk, PETA's Sexiest Vegetarian Over 50, and author of *Live Raw,
Live Raw Around the World,* and *The Ultimate Book of Modern Juicing*

"*The Good Karma Diet* shows you why it's in your self-interest to care about animals and the future of this planet. You feel better and avoid the ills plaguing American society, like heart disease and obesity. We all win a better world. And, good karma is delicious."

—Jane Velez-Mitchell, creator of JaneUnchained.com,
journalist, and author of *Addict Nation*

"Once again, Victoria Moran provides a plan that can help so many people. One of my med school professors taught, 'We kill the cows and the cows kill us.' Moran shows us how good the results can be when 'We cherish all life and life will love you back.'"

—Joel K. Kahn, MD, FACC, Professor of Cardiology, Wayne State University
School of Medicine, and author of *The Whole Heart Solution*

"The secret to happiness is simple: do your best to contribute to more happiness in the lives of others. Let *The Good Karma Diet* be your how-to manual and begin today to create a more joyful life for yourself, others, and the planet."

—**Sharon Gannon**, cofounder of Jivamukti Yoga, and author of
Simple Recipes for Joy

"Inspirational and thought-provoking. A profound and uplifting book that just may save your life."

—**Robert Ostfeld, MD, MSc., FACC,** director of the Cardiac Wellness Program,
Montefiore Medical Center, New York

The
Good Karma
Diet

Also by Victoria Moran

*Main Street Vegan: Everything You Need to Know to
Eat Healthfully and Live Compassionately in the Real World*

The Love-Powered Diet: Eating for Freedom, Health, and Joy

*Living a Charmed Life: Your Guide to Finding Magic
in Every Moment of Every Day*

*Fat, Broke & Lonely No More: Your Personal Solution to Overeating,
Overspending, and Looking for Love in All the Wrong Places*

*Younger by the Day: 365 Ways to Rejuvenate
Your Body and Revitalize Your Spirit*

Fit from Within: 101 Simple Secrets to Change Your Body and Your Life

Lit from Within: A Simple Guide to the Art of Inner Beauty

*Creating a Charmed Life: Sensible, Spiritual Secrets
Every Busy Woman Should Know*

Shelter for the Spirit: Create Your Own Haven in a Hectic World

Get the Fat Out: 501 Simple Ways to Cut the Fat in Any Diet

Compassion the Ultimate Ethic: An Exploration of Veganism

The
Good Karma
Diet

. . . .

Eat Gently, Feel Amazing,
Age in Slow Motion

Victoria Moran

With Recipes from Doris Fin, CHHC, AADP

JEREMY P. TARCHER | PENGUIN
an imprint of Penguin Random House | New York

JEREMY P. TARCHER/PENGUIN
An imprint of Penguin Random House LLC
375 Hudson Street
New York, New York 10014

Most Tarcher/Penguin books are available at special quantity discounts for bulk
purchase for sales promotions, premiums, fund-raising, and educational needs.
Special books or book excerpts also can be created to fit specific needs. For details,
write: SpecialMarkets@penguinrandomhouse.com.

Library of Congress Cataloging-in-Publication Data

Moran, Victoria.
The good karma diet : eat gently, feel amazing, age in slow motion / Victoria Moran ; with recipes
from Doris Fin, CHHC, AADP.
p.   cm.
Includes index.
ISBN 978-0-399-17315-8
1. Vegan cooking.   2. Vegetarianism.   I. Fin, Doris.   II. Title.
RM236.M67   2015
641.5'636—dc23   2015005072

Printed in the United States of America
1   3   5   7   9   10   8   6   4   2

Book design by Gretchen Achilles

Contents

······

Please Read the Introduction   ix

1. My Good Karma Story   1

2. The Good Karma Diet   5

3. Have It Your Way   15

4. Liven Things Up   25

5. High-Green, High-Raw, High-Energy Eating   33

6. 21 Days to Good Health and Good Karma   43

7. Good Cheer and a Good Blender   53

8. Kitchen Contentment   61

9. Skinny Is Skinny. Healthy Is Happy   69

10. The Kitchen Is Closed   77

11. Pummeling Perfectionism   81

12. Before You Feed Yourself, Nourish Yourself   87

13. Put on a Happy Plate   93

14. Numbers and Letters and Science, Oh My!   99

15. Animal Stories   109

16. Do Unto Others   115

17. If Mama Ain't Happy   127

18. Food and Health and Price and Justice   135

19. But Everybody Says Something Different   147

20. Gimme a V!   159

21. Awesome Ancestors   169

22. Plant-Built Muscle   179

23. Beauty, Fashion, and Good Karma Shopping   191

24. The Body Electric   207

25. The Good Karma Life   213

Appendix A: Life Can Be Hard, So Food Should Be Easy Recipes   219

Appendix B: Books for Your Bedside and for Your Kitchen   275

Acknowledgments   281

Index   285

Please Read
the Introduction

......

This is an incredibly important introduction. I feel as if I'm introducing you to the man or woman you just might fall in love with, or to the CEO who's going to make you vice president and richer than you've ever been. I'm introducing you here, of course, not to another human being, but to a remarkable way of life that you may well fall in love with. If you do, you'll know very soon that things have taken a decidedly upward turn. Nothing will ever be the same.

You'll be doing something revolutionary: making food choices based on kindness and love instead of preferences formed in childhood, or opinions about calories, carbs, and fat grams that developed later. Those judgments disregard the law of karma that states that every action (and word and thought, too) has a consequence. If we acted as truly rational beings, we'd take only those actions, dietary and otherwise, that result in positive consequences, the proverbial "happily ever after." But we don't—at least, not all the time.

Karma is a fascinating concept. The word comes from the Sanskrit (it literally means "action"), and this principle of "what goes around comes around" is central to the worldview of spiritual teachings with Indian origins—Hinduism, yoga, Buddhism, Jainism. Sharon Gannon, cofounder of Jivamukti Yoga, explains it: "What we do, no matter how insignificant it may seem, affects everyone else, including ourselves. Our present reality depends on how we have treated others in our past. That's good news because it means we can change what we don't like—our karma—by changing our actions."

And karma isn't exclusively Indian. Jesus expounded on it clearly when he said, ". . . whatsoever a man soweth, that shall he also reap." Even the physical world reflects this postulate. Remember learning in high school Newton's Third Law, "For every action, there is an equal and opposite reaction"? Newton was thinking physics, not that eating peanut butter out of the jar in front of the TV would make us feel bad, but it's fascinating that life on earth is, to a large extent, a ceaseless dance of cause and effect.

What does this have to do with your dinner? Plenty. When you make food choices that you're proud of, that meet your own high standards, the meal will be uniquely satisfying. Of course you'll want it to look and smell and taste good. You'll be sure there's enough of it and enough substance to it that your body and brain will get the message that you ate. It will be in line with what you know about health and nutrition, so you'll feel that you've genuinely done your body good. And it won't have hurt anyone else. You will have done the research to know that the exquisite square of dark chocolate putting a perfect period at the end of your meal didn't come from slave labor, as a great deal of chocolate does. And you'll know that no sentient being suffered or died in order for you to nourish yourself.

"So that's the catch," you might be thinking. "Vegan propaganda!" (Definitions: vegetarian = no meat or fish; vegan = no animal products of any kind, including dairy products and eggs.) Let me come clean at the outset: I can't even envision a diet connected with good karma that includes animal foods. Can somebody be healthy and eat some meat and eggs and dairy products? Of course. Unless someone is dealing with heart disease or kidney disease or gout, conditions known to be directly impacted by the consumption of animal protein and fat, the body can handle some animal foods. I don't say this as a health professional—I'm not one—but as an observer of life.

However, I contend that only a vegan meal is capable of producing in the person who consumes it the deepest level of well-being, satisfaction that comes without any glimmer of conscious or unconscious guilt. Only a vegan can honestly look a cow, pig, sheep, turkey, or chicken in the eye. Fishes count, too. It was while observing them that Franz Kafka commented, "Now I can look at you in peace; I don't eat you anymore."

Nothing fills us with deep and lasting joy the way that doing a good turn for someone else does. Saving somebody's life, human or animal, is that "good turn" in spades, and you can start precisely where you are. I don't expect you to go from zero to Moby in nothing flat, but I invite you to consider the possibility that nothing will more readily bring about a state of peace with your body and your food than making sure no one else's body *is* your food.

Upping the Radiance Factor

When I ventured veganward more than thirty years ago, doing this was (1) really weird and (2) really healthy, because there were almost no vegan junk foods or convenience foods. We ate vegetables, fruits, whole grains, beans, and nuts and seeds almost exclusively. New vegans routinely lost weight (I dropped the final fifty of a sixty-pound excess after making the switch, and it's still gone). Even though we'd never heard of antioxidants, and the first brave soul to put greens in a smoothie had yet to surface, everybody seemed to either take up a sport or adopt twins because we had unbelievable energy. In those days, being vegan protected a person from baked goods. And ice cream. And pizza.

Those protections are no longer in place. There are vegan versions of nearly every snack food and comfort food known to humankind, and that's good. We'll save more animals when potential vegans don't have to fear the loss of chicken-like nuggets. Nevertheless, if you want to dazzle onlookers with your state of health and the way you look now and as time goes by, you'll need a more enlightened take on food and self-care. You'll be heading toward "vegan with lots of produce and minimal cupcakes." And you'll get to grow into it at your own pace.

The Good Karma Diet, which is, in all honesty, the Good Karma Life, is a process of moving from doing fine to doing splendidly, or from not so healthy and not so happy to vibrant health and the unshakeable conviction that there's a miracle hiding in this day somewhere and you're going to find it. It puts you in harmony with the needs of your body and the calling of your spirit. It's living in a way that requires you to treat yourself like the divine being you are, and eating in a way that lets you choose from foods that are as beautiful as you yourself have ever wished to be.

This way of living and eating has been around awhile—some would say since the Garden of Eden—and it has a growing body of admirers and adherents, with some celebrities and illuminati sprinkling glitter on its reputation. Right now, however, the only person who matters is you, learning what you need to and getting as much support as you require to do this joyously and successfully from now until forever.

If you stick with me on this, you cannot fail. Nothing is perfect except the spirit within you and the Power that got you here. Everything else, including the choices you make about eating and exercise and the rest, is an attempt to replicate that love and beauty and energy. The closer you come, the more incredible you'll feel. And on days when you're not as close as you'd like to be, that essence of you is still perfect, and that Power loves you as much as ever. Unlike old-fashioned diets characterized by on and off, or lose and gain, this is an invitation to live a more momentous life than most people believe is possible. It is a gateway to a growth experience that will get richer and deeper and more magnificent as you go along.

I'm offering you an opportunity to upgrade the way you eat, live, see yourself, and relate to those around you. You can expect to lose weight if you have weight to lose. You'll find yourself waking up in a good mood more often. Your skin will have that luminous look that bespeaks health and clean living. And you'll get compliments.

You may overcome a pesky health complaint. People who nourish themselves with plant foods—mostly whole and unprocessed, with a lot of salads, fresh fruits, colorful smoothies, and green juices in the mix—report leaving behind everything from IBS (irritable bowel syndrome) to eczema, depression to migraines. I can't tell you how your body, mind, and spirit will work together to heal some specific ailment. If you have medical concerns, you'll want to work with a reputable health care provider, ideally one who is open to this way of eating, and chart together what improvements you're making, and what medications can be decreased or eliminated.

Dealing with pathologies is beyond the scope of this book, and I'm not recommending self-diagnosis or self-treatment. If you're under a doctor's care, consult with him or her about what you intend to do and proceed with that guidance. (To find a compatible physician in your area, check out VegDocs.com.) Everyone else, start today!

Getting the Most from This Book

Are you excited yet? Either way, that's fine for now, because I'm excited enough for both of us. I'm excited that you'll be healthier, but I'm more excited that you'll be happier. Happy people do healthy things. Customize your Good Karma journey to your own life and circumstances. If you've tried something similar before and it didn't seem to work for you, give this a shot. You wouldn't be in this philosophical neighborhood again if there weren't something here for you.

In addition to this book's twenty-five chapters, you'll find sprinkled throughout "Good Karma Stories," vignettes from men and women whose lives changed for the very-much-better as a result of altering their food choices. In some cases, this looks like pure cause and effect, i.e., they lost weight or got healthier as a result of their dietary changes. More often, the good karma is more far-reaching. It's a whole-life turnaround ignited not only by eating whole foods but also by realizing the dignity and essential worth of every being who has, or had, life on earth and the desire to keep it. In addition, you'll find here and there *Good Karma Tips* (*GKTs*) that offer practical suggestions you can start to implement right now.

While this is a living book, not a cookbook, you will, nevertheless, find as Appendix A "Life Can Be Hard, So Food Should Be Easy Recipes," from Toronto recipe creator, culinary photographer, and raw food chef Doris Fin, CHHC, AADP. These recipes are beautiful and easy to make, and Doris's style of food prep—very fresh, very colorful, mostly raw—makes for the instant karma of feeling amazing not long after you swallow. You don't need to become a full-time "raw fooder"—I haven't done that—but the more alive the food you eat, the more alive you'll look and feel.

In Appendix B, you'll find suggestions for books to read, and some with which to cook, after you finish this one. Books are the great renewers, connecting you again and again with the passion you feel when a novel idea first ignites your imagination.

I also wanted to insert a note for anyone who follows my work and knows that this is not my first book with "diet" in the title. You might be wondering how many diets one woman is entitled to come up with! Here's the explanation: that earlier book, *The Love-Powered Diet*, is about overcoming food addiction; it gives any reader dealing with compulsive eating a way to restructure from the inside out. It also suggests and details a vegan foodstyle, just as this book does, but *The Good Karma Diet* is designed to appeal to everyone, not just people who have had an unusually troublesome relationship with food. This book also leans toward a high-green, high-raw, youth-preserving way of eating that I had not fully discovered when I wrote my other "diet" book.

So, here we are: poised to sparkle and shine, to feel exquisitely alive, and to make a genuine difference in this world. I'm humbled and grateful that you're trusting me as a guide on your journey. I honor where you've already been and what you already know, which I'm betting is considerable. I promise to tell you the truth as I see it, recognizing that others may see it differently. And I'll tell you what I do myself, because it is apparently working.

There's no need to overhaul your life overnight, but don't dawdle, either. You're offered something here that goes far beyond the soulless rhetoric of the weight loss industry, the food giants, and the "Oh, dear, dear, we mustn't be too radical" nutritional establishment. We're not talking about doing a little better and feeling a little better, but rather about regeneration. It starts in your kitchen but it expands to touch every aspect of your life. This is dietary yoga, transformation for body and soul. If these ideas resonate with you and you're ready to make this shift, you're in for a divinely delicious adventure.

The
Good Karma
Diet

1

......

My Good Karma Story

didn't know it was possible to feel this good.

I woke up not long ago thinking, "This is the craziest thing: if I had a real job, I'd be retiring this year, and yet I feel more alive and more energized than when I was twenty." I knew it was what Arnold Ehret, a nineteenth-century "food reformer," had called "Paradise Health." I had it, physically and emotionally.

I'd been on a pretty good path for a long time. Although I spent the first thirty years of my life bingeing and dieting—always gaining or losing weight, and conversely losing and gaining my flimsy self-esteem—I finally got so tired of that un-merry merry-go-round that I gave up the fight and was open to recovery from the inside out. Food was my drug, so I went to meetings like any other addict. I put my appetite in the hands of God, and God gave me my life back, only better.

Once I wasn't eating for a fix anymore, I was able to move toward plant-based eating, and despite fits and starts and goofs and lapses, I ultimately ended up at profound, committed veganism—nothing from an animal, not fish or low-fat yogurt or eggs, even when hidden in a banana-walnut muffin.

I made the veg choice, as Isaac Bashevis Singer said that he, too, had done "for the health of the chickens." I knew a little of the horrors of factory farming, and that even small, local farmers, as dedicated as they are to doing things better, are caught up in the economic necessity of having to separate mother dairy cows from their babies and sending the unneeded boy calves off for veal. Small farms acquire the chicks who will be laying hens from the same hatcheries that serve factory farms and ruthlessly kill the boy babies shortly after they break free from their shells. And, of course, the slaughterhouse ends things for all farmed animals, usually while they're still young.

With my vegan conversion, it was easy to keep the weight off and avoid the heart disease and diabetes that plague both sides of my family of origin. I raised a beautiful vegan daughter, Adair, wrote several books, and enjoyed some breathtaking moments of speaking for large audiences and going on TV. I had trials like everyone else, and even some tragedies. My first husband, Patrick Moran, suffered from an anxiety disorder and took his life when our daughter was only four. In 2007, my sixteen-year-old stepson, James Melton, died from a freak illness. These were devastating experiences, to be sure, and yet, like everyone else who loved Patrick and James, I muddled through.

But life likes pushing us to more and better, and a few years ago I felt the nudge to clean things up. Less food made in factories and more that grew in dirt. Less delivery food, even though I live in New York City, where delivery is an inalienable right. And a higher percentage of raw food—not slavishly or fanatically (as a compulsive overeater with a daily reprieve, I don't do well with fads and tangents); but my soul or my cells or something deep inside pressed me to take this turn. And so much is better because of it.

It used to be that when people asked, "How are you?" I'd say, "I'm okay." And that was true. Unless I'd picked up a cold or pulled a muscle at the gym, I was absolutely okay. Now I say, "I'm fabulous." And today that's true. Of course, I can still get a cold or pull a muscle or feel dramatically down when something disappointing happens, but my overarching sense of how it feels to live today in this body is some kind of wonderful. The only thing that's changed is that the food I eat today comes in brighter colors with less packaging. And I use my juicer and blender every single day.

Fresh foods—vegetables, fruits, nuts, seeds, and sprouts—are my mainstays; and I look to legumes and whole grains for concentrated protein and a money-saving, low-fat way to get the safe and satisfied feeling that comes from something warm and hearty. I eat more cooked foods in winter, more raw foods in summer.

The approach detailed in chapter 5, "High-Green, High-Raw, High-Energy Eating," is, to my mind, the best of all dietary worlds—and it's doable by mere mortals. People can be tyrannical with themselves about their food choices, but life is too glorious a gift for that. Swami Vivekananda, the first Indian yogi to travel to America way back in the 1890s, said, "Don't make your kitchen your church." Good plan.

The first thing I noticed after making the switch to more fresh food was how positive I felt. Greater contentment showed up even before energy and strength and clarity, but those have come, too. Strangers tell me nice things—that I have good skin or good posture or that I look younger than my age. Now, I know we're talking vegetables, not miracles, but the aging process is slower than I'd expected. I find that green juices, exercise, eight hours of sleep, regular meditation, and adventures invite youthfulness. And lethargy, worry, getting stuck in ruts, and eating too many manufactured foods exacerbate the negative aspects of age. (There are positive aspects to later life, by the way. Learning how to live can take some time, but once you get it down, it can be pretty fabulous.)

Empty-nesters at this point, my husband, William, and I live with our rescue dog, Forbes (his name is a reminder that the greatest wealth comes from those we love), and we both work from home. Our children—Adair, and William's daughter, Siân, and son, Erik—are making their way uniquely and creatively in the world. I'm blessed to be able to write about what I believe in, travel as much as I can stand,

and host an Internet radio show that allows me to converse in depth with people I respect and admire.

I also have a bouncing baby business, something I never dreamed would be part of my destiny. It's Main Street Vegan Academy, an in-person immersion course that trains and certifies Vegan Lifestyle Coaches and Educators (VLCEs). There are now alumni in nine countries and I'm proud as punch of each one of them. They're part of a far larger vegan community with which I feel honored and lucky to be associated. This is a movement toward unprecedented compassion, greater health for more people, and, because of the environmental issues gravely exacerbated by animal agriculture, catastrophe-averting good sense. Being part of a groundswell this momentous is, as far as I can tell, about as good as it gets.

2

......

The Good Karma Diet

Good Karma eating is as simple as can be: comprise your meals of plants instead of animals and, most of the time, choose unprocessed plant foods, meaning that they got from the garden or orchard or field to your kitchen with minimal corporate interference. This way of choosing foods is not the norm in our society, but it is what comes naturally to us.

Harvey Diamond, coauthor of the 1980s mega-seller *Fit for Life*, used to challenge his audiences with: "If you give a small child a bunny and an apple, and she eats the bunny and plays with the apple, I'll buy you a car." I've always loved this because it's so obvious: deep inside, we know that animals are friends and that fruit—and vegetables and grains and beans and nuts and seeds—are food. Accept that, and act on it, and you've got yourself a Good Karma Diet.

Right off the bat, this way of eating gives you good karma in two distinct but complementary ways. The first is self-explanatory: by eating foods of high nutrient density and avoiding the animal products and processed foods that your body can have trouble dealing with, you'll reap the rewards of improved health. The second is a bit more mystical: you do good and you get good back.

As is true for life in general, it's probably better to do this with unselfish motives than with rewards in mind, but even if your motivation is to become thinner, healthier, or more youthful, you'll be doing something modestly heroic at the same time. This way of eating and living could, with enough people doing it, lessen the suffering of billions of animals. I know it's hard to think in terms of billions, but if you imagine counting the *individual beings* one at a time, you get some of the impact. In addition, 98 percent of the animals raised for food suffer horrifically on factory farms before being slaughtered. Every time you eat a vegan meal, you're voting for something different.

This choice also lightens the burden on the planet. Raising animals for food in the numbers we do today calls for an exorbitant amount of water and fossil fuels. It leads to vast "lagoons" of animal waste, and the release into the atmosphere of tons of greenhouse gases, mostly in the form of methane. (Chapter 17, "If Mama Ain't Happy," goes into more detail.)

In addition, we've known since Frances Moore Lappé's *Diet for a Small Planet* back in the 1970s that eating plant foods ourselves, instead of raising grain and soybeans to feed animals destined for slaughter, can make more food available for hungry people around the globe. And the yogis knew three thousand years ago that eating as a vegetarian was conducive to spiritual growth and inner peace. Moreover, by simply living your life and shining your light—this includes not coming off as preachy or superior—you'll inspire others to get healthier and open their hearts to more compassion.

What you have here is holistic dining at its finest, with body and soul onboard. Eating whole, plant foods is scientifically validated as being both nutritionally adequate and anti-pathological. In other words, it cures stuff. Not everything. But reversal of such scourges as coronary disease and type 2 diabetes among people on this kind of diet has been repeatedly reported in the scientific literature; and the preventive potential of this way of eating is supported by ample research. (Michael Greger, MD, follows the publication in credible journals worldwide of studies related to nutrition and health; he reports on these in short daily videos on his site, NutritionFacts.org, and sends them without charge to subscribers.)

Making It Happen

If this sounds great but going all the way seems impossible right now, go partway. Americans' consumption of animal foods has, as I write this, been decreasing annually for several years, primarily because non-vegans are making vegan choices some—or much—of the time. They fix a veggie burger or black beans and rice, or they order their latté with soy, or have a green smoothie for breakfast so they'll look prettier and—what do you know? The statistics get prettier, too.

GKT

A bring-along emergency kit for Good Karma diners might be an apple, a bag of raw nuts, and some high-cacao-content dark chocolate. These are easy to transport lest you find yourself in a food desert.

Whether you're going vegan today or taking an incremental approach, you'll start to intercept cruelty and killing from day one. Every step in this direction—doing Meatless Mondays, or eating vegan before six p.m., as food journalist Mark Bittman's book title *VB6* suggests—is important and powerful. Just keep moving forward. Here's a sample step-by-step plan that does the job within a year:

- **January 1**—*As of today, I no longer consume chickens and eggs.* (This includes the invisible eggs in conventional cookies, pancakes, etc.) Once you cut out chickens and eggs, you're a hero, saving the lives of birds—birds who can recognize flock members and humans, birds who can know their own names when someone cares enough to give them one. How many? "An average American meat-eater is responsible for the death of twenty-eight meat chickens, one laying hen, and one discarded male chick every year," says Nick Cooney, author of *Veganomics.* See: you're a lifesaver and you just got started.

- **May 1**—*As of today, I eat no fishes.* Sometimes you'll hear someone say, "I'm vegetarian, but I eat fish." A fish is not a vegetable. Fish can indeed feel pain, a fact documented repeatedly by recent science. "Fish are fast learners with a keen sense of time," says Mary Finelli, director of FishFeel .org. "They recognize other individuals, can keep track of complex social relationships, and work cooperatively with other species." You'll save the lives of fishes when you stop eating them, obviously, but you started this process when you stopped eating chickens, because fish meal is a large part of the feed given to chickens and other farmed animals. When you make it to vegetarian (eating no animals), you'll save a substantial 225 fishes per year. (This number was calculated from government statistics for the intriguing blog CountingAnimals.com, "a place for people who love animals and numbers.")

- **September 1**—*As of today, I eat no flesh of any kind.* Congratulations: you're a vegetarian. Like Albert Schweitzer and Benjamin Spock, Charlotte Brontë and Harriet Beecher Stowe, Ellen DeGeneres and Paul McCartney, you have opted not to eat anybody who had a face. You're in good company. If you miss the texture, flavor, or dinnertime ritual of certain meats, there are high-quality veggie-meats out there from companies including Beyond Meat, Field Roast, Gardein, and Tofurky.

- **December 1**—*As of today, I ingest no dairy products.* By now, this should be easy. You already may be making your own nut milks, or the place in your fridge where the cow's milk used to be is now reserved for soy or rice or almond or coconut milk. Sold in most supermarkets, these are low in calories and equal to or higher in calcium content than cow's milk. If you haven't checked out the commercial nondairy cheeses, try them. Daiya melts and is ideal for pizza; Miyoko's Kitchen and Treeline are gourmet dairy-free cheese brands you could proudly offer a French person. Or try your hand at making your own cheeses, cheese spreads, and cheese sauces with the recipes in *Artisan Vegan Cheese,* by Miyoko Schinner, and *The Cheesy Vegan,* by John Schlimm.

Once the dairy products are gone, you're likely to feel amazing. In fact, if you're prone to fatigue, congestion, allergy symptoms, frequent colds, or GI upsets, you might want to let go of dairy milk, cheese, and yogurt *first.* It's anecdotal, but many people report relief from such ailments as soon as they part ways with what Michael Klaper, MD, likes to call "baby cow growth formula." But isn't milk nature's perfect food? Yes—for calves. The majority of humans—and the vast majority of those of African or Asian descent—don't tolerate it well at all.

Once you're fully vegan, celebrate! The only thing you need to "do" nutritionally is take a vitamin B_{12} supplement of about 100 micrograms a day as a tiny, tasty, melt-in-your mouth tablet. B_{12} is not reliably found in plant foods unless they've been fortified with it, and a lack of B_{12} is dangerous.

You'll read more on this in chapter 14, "Numbers and Letters and Science, Oh My!" This single missing element in a plant-food diet pains many vegans. If this is the perfect diet, it ought to be, well, *perfect*. But this is life on earth: extraordinary, magnificent, and absolutely not perfect. Bacteria in our mouths and intestines do make some B_{12}, and maybe at some point in evolutionary history we all made enough, just as our long-ago ancestors made their own vitamin C and now we don't. I look at taking B_{12} as a tiny surcharge for the privilege of being vegan.

Yes You Can

Phasing out animal foods is the most important aspect of Good Karma Diet. If you hear yourself saying "I could never give up ice cream" (or something else), realize that you may just be short on *vegucation*. There are lots of rich, luscious nondairy ice creams on the market, and you can make exquisite homemade ice cream, both vegan and raw, with only a DIY gene and an ice cream maker.

GKT

Be prepped and ready. If you're eating a lot of raw food, you'll probably want to shop twice a week to keep sufficient fresh foods on hand.

If you have the necessary information and you're still saying "I could never give up . . . ," listen to yourself. You're affirming weakness. There you are, created, the Bible says, in the image and likeness of God, and you're brought to your knees by a scoop of French vanilla.

You're bigger than that. You can eat plants and save lives. You can give your life exponentially more meaning by living in a way that decreases suffering just because you got up and chose a kind breakfast.

Without this commitment, the Good Karma Diet would be, as much as I hate to say it, just a diet. To me, a diet is: "Eat this and don't eat that, and feel guilty when you screw up, which of course you will because you're only human, for heaven's sake, and nobody can be on a diet forever." That doesn't really make you want to say, "I'll have what she's having."

But understand and embrace the compassion piece, the soul-deep conviction that you're here to make life easier for others, regardless of species; and then everything else—whatever tweaks you might make because of an allergy, a digestive peculiarity, a personal preference—will come with little effort. This lifts that word "diet" from the deprivational depths and restores its original meaning from the Greek *diaita*, "a way of life." And this particular way of life is one replete with meaning and fulfillment and joy.

Brenda's Good Karma Story

The year was 1978. I was a first-year nutrition student and an omnivore fascinated by vegetarianism, the topic of today's lecture. Our professor spent ten minutes teaching future dietitians all we would learn about vegetarian diets while attending university: that vegetarian diets with dairy products and eggs were risky, and pure vegetarian (vegan) diets downright dangerous.

I began my career as a public health nutritionist, espousing the benefits of the Four Food Groups; yet every time the "v-word" appeared in the scientific literature, my heart skipped a beat. There was something attractive about a diet driven by compassion. Many childhood memories were of animal encounters—moving worms from sidewalk to grass, talking to turtles, and passionately cheering for the bull at a horrific bullfight in Spain. Somehow, even with all my "knowledge" about the "necessity" of meat and dairy, these products were being squeezed out of my own diet by lentils and tofu.

In 1989, a friend who was an avid hunter stopped by for coffee before a hunting trip. I asked him how he could feel good about pulling the trigger on a defenseless animal. I asked him if killing made him feel like more of a man. His response changed the course of my life. "You have no right to criticize me," he said. "Just because you don't have the guts to pull the trigger doesn't mean you're not responsible for its being pulled, every time you buy a piece of meat camouflaged in cellophane. You're simply paying someone else to do the dirty work for you. And at least the deer I eat had a life. I doubt you can say the same for the animals on your plate."

I was silenced. I knew it was time to take responsibility for my food choices. What I learned filled me with shame, guilt, and outrage, but most important, it reconnected me with the animals I so mindlessly called food.

I faced some interesting personal and professional challenges. A young mom in Northern Ontario where vegetarians were as rare as Bigfoot, I was uncertain how my husband, Paul, would respond when I asked if he'd be willing to nix meat and dairy. Even though his closest friend was the deer hunter, he said, "I thought you'd never ask." He always was a step ahead of me.

I considered changing careers. How could I, in good conscience, teach people that we need meat for protein and milk for calcium, and yet how could I avoid it when all our nutrition education materials were founded on these principles? I didn't know any other vegetarians, and wondered if I was the only vegetarian dietitian on the planet. I imagined being forcibly ousted from the profession. But if I didn't stand up for what I believed in, I risked betraying my own conscience.

Twenty-five years have passed. I did not leave my profession, and I learned that I have many vegetarian and vegan colleagues within it. I've written nine books on plant-based nutrition, published four peer-reviewed journal articles, and I've spoken at professional conferences around the world. I am the lead dietitian in groundbreaking research on plant-based diets and on diabetes in the Marshall Islands, and a past chair of the Vegetarian Nutrition Dietetic Practice Group of the American Dietetic Association (now the Academy of Nutrition and Dietetics). When I think of how fear could so easily have shifted the course of my career, and my life, I am profoundly grateful that courage and conscience prevailed, allowing my life to unfold so naturally.

—**Brenda Davis**, Registered Dietitian, lecturer, and author of
Becoming Vegan. BrendaDavisRD.com

3

......

Have It Your Way

There are as many ways to eat a vegan diet as there are people who discover it. Just about any way you do it, provided you focus on unprocessed foods, include vitamin B_{12}, and make a few adjustments for your individual needs and preferences, can be viable and health-promoting.

Most people start by eating the same sorts of meals they're used to, simply replacing animal foods with plant foods, i.e., scrambled tofu instead of scrambled eggs, plant meat—Tofurky sausages, Gardein sliders—instead of animal meat, or a veggie burrito or burger or stir-fry instead of the *con carne* version. Eventually, most of us move away from believing that every meal needs something resembling the foods we're no longer eating, and we let delicious dishes made from vegetables, beans, whole grains, nuts, and seeds take on the entrée role.

While most vegans are free spirits and don't follow a single dietary philosophy, there are "denominations" within veganism and near-veganism, and I'll outline them here. If you don't care about such distinctions, they're not essential for your making a start. The various approaches are far more alike than different, each stressing the importance of natural, minimally processed plant foods. I personally am in awe of and in debt to the people behind each one.

The Whole-Food, Plant-Based Diet (WFPB)

The whole-food, plant-based diet (WFPB) is the popular term coined by nutritional biochemist T. Colin Campbell, PhD, lead researcher of the China Study, the largest population-based nutritional study ever conducted. In *The Low-Carb Fraud*, Dr. Campbell and Howard Jacobson, PhD, define the WFPB diet as: "whole foods . . . as close to their natural state as possible. A wide variety of fruits, vegetables, grains, nuts, and seeds make up the bulk of the diet. It includes no refined products, such as white sugar or white flour; no additives, preservatives, or other chemical concoctions . . . no refined fat, including olive or coconut oils; and minimal—or better yet, no—consumption of animal products, perhaps 0 to 5 percent of total calories at most."

The Starch Solution

John McDougall, MD, a California internist who's devoted his career to healing people from the chronic diseases of Western civilization, takes a very low-fat approach and celebrates the basic starches—rice, wheat, potatoes, barley, taro, and so forth—that have supported humanity for eons. Vegetables, fruits, and beans comprise the rest of the diet. He named a book for this: *The Starch Solution*.

The Esselstyn Approach

The Cleveland Clinic research study done by Caldwell Esselstyn Jr., MD, showed how an oil-free, whole-food, plant-exclusive diet with plenty of greens was capable of reversing heart disease in patients whose cardiologists could no longer help them. He expounds on his long-term study and its results in his book *Prevent and Reverse Heart Disease*.

His son Rip, a handsome endurance athlete and former fire-fighter, takes the same approach and calls it "plant-strong" in his books, *The Engine 2 Diet* and *My Beef with Meat*. (The Campbell and Esselstyn plans are virtually identical, and the McDougall plan is very similar, all emphasizing whole, plant foods and no oil. This way of eating was showcased in the popular documentary and subsequent best-selling book *Forks over Knives*.)

The Nutritarian Diet

Joel Fuhrman, MD, author of the *New York Times* best-seller *Eat to Live*, recommends a "nutritarian" diet built primarily around vegetables, fruits, and legumes. Whole grains are allowed, but not emphasized, and moderate consumption of nuts and seeds is encouraged. He suggests getting at least 90 percent of calories from whole plant foods, leaving up to 10 percent for the occasional indulgence and for animal products for those who aren't going to part with them entirely. In my practice as a health counselor I found that clients did well with this approach that emphasizes "nutrient density," getting the most nutrition for every calorie.

GKT

Eat Dr. Joel Fuhrman's "G-Bombs" every day. The author of *Never Diet Again* ensures a nutritional head start with Greens, Beans, Onions, Mushrooms, Berries, and Seeds—true super-foods that boast major antioxidant power. In the laboratory, plain old white mushrooms gobbled up cancer cells like nobody's business.

Plant-Based, Lower-Carb

A newer player on the vegan field is a higher-protein, higher-fat, lower-carbohydrate rendition of a way of eating that is still, by definition, high in naturally occurring carbohydrate because that is the nutritive property that predominates in most plant foods. If you've read a lot of diet books, this sounds bad ("The carbs are coming! Run for the hills!"), but it's actually good. We're designed to function on a diet that derives most of its calories from the carbohydrates in unrefined plant foods. Attempting to avoid all carbohydrates because refined sugar and white bread aren't good for you would be like avoiding marriage because some men beat their wives.

Despite the profusion of laboratory and epidemiological studies supporting the efficacy of the approaches outlined earlier, some people feel that they do better with a little more protein and fat. Their predilection was given scientific backup by David J. A. Jenkins, MD, PhD (he developed the concept of the glycemic index), who devised a plant-based diet favoring non-starchy vegetables, soy foods and mock meats, lower-carb beans (mung, great northern, lima, fava), nuts, seeds, and avocado, and low-sugar fruits, such as berries. This diet has been called "Eco Atkins."

Ellen Jaffe Jones and Alan Roettinger take a similar approach in their book, *Paleo Vegan*, emphasizing unprocessed foods and designed to bring about some meeting of the minds between the high-protein/low-carb paleo diet folks and those of us who wish to keep animals off our plates.

Macrobiotics

The macrobiotic diet appeals to those who find that unrefined carbohydrates, including a plentitude of grains, make them feel physically and mentally in tune and on target. While macrobiotics, with its Japanese heritage, traditionally includes some fish, it can easily be vegan (see *The Kind Diet*, by Alicia Silverstone). The fundamental precept is to maintain a balance of yin and yang energies, achieved through a diet based on whole grains, brown rice in particular, beans, including soy, local vegetables and sea vegetables, fermented foods such as miso (soy-based soup base and seasoning) and shoyu (natural soy sauce), and a little fruit, often baked or stewed, while avoiding refined foods and most raw foods.

Ayurveda

Ayurveda is a healing tradition from India that translates as "science of life." Popularized in the West by Deepak Chopra's book *Perfect Health*, it includes more than diet but has much to say on the subject.

Because it's Indian and evolved alongside yoga, its dietary suggestions are basically vegetarian but traditionally include milk, cheese, and ghee (clarified butter), used both for cooking and medicinal purposes. Many contemporary practitioners and adherents of Ayurveda are vegan. (*The Ayurvedic Vegan Kitchen*, by Talya Lutzker, is a useful guide.)

There is no single Ayurvedic diet because the philosophy cites three body types—Vata, Pitta, and Kapha, and combinations of these—each requiring different foods and means of food preparation. For example, thin, flighty Vata becomes "spaced out" from too many greens and raw vegetables, but can eat these with the addition of oil, seen as heavy and grounding. Depending on body type, foods favored in Ayurveda include lentils, split mung dal, and split peas; rice and barley; citrus and other fruits; nuts, especially blanched almonds; vegetables of all kinds; and spices, emphasizing those commonly used in India: turmeric, cardamom, cinnamon, ginger, and fennel.

The Raw Food Diet

Proponents of raw food and high-raw diets include Gabriel Cousens, MD (*Raw Food Works*) and Kris Carr (*Crazy Sexy Diet*), who emphasize the healing and detoxifying properties of fresh, raw vegetables and sprouts, fruits, nuts and seeds, fermented foods (sauerkraut, kimchi, fermented nut cheeses), freshly extracted juices, and smoothies, often green.

Raw food can be straightforward and therapeutic, illustrated by the beautiful but simple meals served at healing centers such as the Ann Wigmore Institute, Hippocrates Health Institute, Optimal Health Institutes, and Tree of Life. Also on the raw culinary continuum is the rich, gourmet cuisine that draws rave reviews and an enthusiastic clientele to five-star raw restaurants around the world.

People who eat raw most of the time tend to save the more elaborate dishes, often nut-based and high in fat, for social gatherings and special occasions.

I believe that if you were to adopt any one of the ways of eating described here, or some combination of them, you'd be doing yourself, not to mention the animals and the earth, a great favor. All these plans have in common the elimination or severe reduction of not only animal foods but also processed, fragmented foods, and the recommendation to eat plenty of whole plant foods—no skimping, no deprivation. The Good Karma Diet, as presented in this book, is high-raw and draws from these other schools of thought as well. This way of eating is sustainable across time, and it produces extremely attractive old people.

Call me shallow, but what better dietary assessment tool could a layperson have than to look at how a diet affects those who've been doing it for an extended period? If a large number of people eating in one way or another are ravishing in their fifties, radiant in their sixties, and robust in their seventies, I'd say they're onto something. I'm not presenting this as scientific fact, or suggesting that people on this type of diet are the only ones who age well. Nevertheless, what I've observed for more than forty years now is that people who have for some time eaten a plant-exclusive diet that includes an abundance of raw fruits and vegetables and freshly extracted juices seem to know where the spigot is to the fountain of youth.

I include in these observations women such as Mimi Kirk, who won "PETA's Sexiest Vegetarian over 50" contest when she was seventy, and Annette Larkins, a YouTube phenomenon who, at seventy-three and without any surgery, looks like a well-preserved forty-five. Cherie Soria, director of the Living Light Culinary Institute in Fort Bragg, California, is in this group: she looks forty from the front and seventeen from the rear (she's sixty-seven). And Karyn Calabrese, Chicago restaurateur and author, has a face and figure that very nearly stop traffic (year of birth: 1942).

It's not just women, either: Dr. Fred Bisci is eighty-five years old and a longtime raw vegan. He still practices as a nutritionist, runs and bikes along the beach on Staten Island, and regularly engages in qigong. When I see these people and others like them—and I know most of them in real life, where Photoshop isn't an issue—I'm witnessing flesh-and-blood evidence of Emerson's words: "Health and beauty are nature's gifts for living by her laws." Because I want what they have, I'm willing to do what they do, to the extent that it's feasible for me. If you want that, too, chapter 4 will detail what we can do to liven things up.

Alan's Good Karma Story

Mine is a charmed life. Wonderful things just keep happening to me. Not that I have recognized every single occurrence as a good thing at the time—I've had as much difficulty seeing through loss, pain, and sorrow as the next guy—but the events in my life have consistently conspired to make everything turn out for the best.

I had some reputation in the culinary world as a private chef and recipe creator, but seven years ago my publisher gave me a project that hurled me on a trajectory I could never have predicted: a book of vegan recipes that could be made in thirty minutes or less. At the time, I enjoyed eating everything, so I had to read up on what exactly vegans ate (which I thought of as what vegans *didn't* eat). As it happened, only tempeh and seitan were unfamiliar. I would be free to use all the ingredients I had always worked with, minus the meat, eggs, and dairy. I was well accustomed to being given strict parameters by my millionaire clients, and this was an unusually liberal set of restraints. That project became the book *Speed Vegan*.

Around this time, my doctor announced that he was putting me on a statin because my cholesterol count was on a ruinous upward arc. I knew a little about statins (and doctors). Everything I had been reading and thinking about coalesced in that moment, and I countered that I had a better idea: I was going on a strict vegan diet. He was incredulous, but it worked. Almost within days, my LDL was in free fall. Some might call that "good karma," but it was only common sense.

I've learned in my life to pay attention to what I feel at least as much as what I think. Even so, I was utterly unprepared for what, in retrospect, was an obvious outcome. I realized that I had always felt a compunction about dining at the expense of sentient creatures, but had suppressed it, as I imagine many people must. The sense of relief at no longer needing to tacitly justify eating animals to myself was profound.

My epiphany was met by a network of some of the friendliest people I've ever encountered, all eager to help me succeed as an author. Doors opened for me. At an age when many people begin to think about ending the working period of their lives, I'm now beginning in earnest. I've come to see my role in a new light. I want to make a significant positive impact on the way people view themselves, as reflected through what they eat. We are—we have the potential to be—sublime creatures, and the food choices we make reflect an important aspect of our success as human beings. It's about what we choose to accept, what we willingly become as a consequence of what we eat, and what that says about us. I want to help facilitate a paradigm shift from unconscious default choices to deliberate heartfelt choices.

As a private chef, I was able to witness power, wealth, and fame up close, and they never impressed me. On the other hand, what has never failed to impress me is kindness. When someone is kind, it shows me what our potential is. It's an inspiring, beautiful sight. Becoming kind is the best sort of karma I could ever imagine, and now it's happening to me.

—**Alan Roettinger**, chef, author of *Extraordinary Vegan*, and coauthor of *Paleo Vegan*. AlanRoettinger.com

4

······

Liven Things Up

When my daughter, Adair, was a tween and teen, we devoted two weeks every summer to eating only raw food: fruits, salads, crudités, and sprouts; dressings, dips, pâtés, and cheeses made from nuts and seeds; vegetable juices and creamy smoothies. When a friend asked her why we did it, she said, "Because everyone deserves to be gorgeous at least two weeks a year." She was talking about the clear eyes, luminous skin, and well-known "glow" that come from eating fresh, raw foods.

But wait a minute: everyone deserves to be gorgeous all year long, every day and every decade. This is what happens with Good Karma dining, upgraded with lots of color (much of it green) and fresh foods that have never seen a processing plant or a cooking pot. Impressive results show up quickly: weight loss, plenty of steady energy, a rested look so people ask if you've been on vacation. You're eating foods that grew. Foods that are, for the most part, in season, so they're fresh and nourish you right now. Foods with vivid colors that don't start with "FDC#."

The phytochemicals and overall nutrient density of greens, berries, fresh juices, and other unheated plant foods can take you light-years beyond a typical, mostly cooked diet that includes lots of packaged and convenience foods, even when you're eating vegan or close to it. (People who've tried that and didn't like it can try *this* and see what happens.)

The color and liveliness of raw food has long appealed to me. I recall an incident, only a couple of years into being vegan. I was in my kitchen making dinner and some prep-ahead dishes for later in the week. They represented the monochromatic fare nearly everyone with an interest in natural foods was eating back then: brown rice and brown bread, lentil soup and onion soup, walnut loaf and wheat germ cutlets. My husband called and asked what I was doing. I replied, "Killing food—uh, I mean, cooking food." With a slip deserving of Dr. Freud, I'd stated where my heart was in terms of bodily sustenance, although I didn't know what to do with this information.

I was aware even then that there were people who ate mostly raw, but they were the ascetics of the vegetarian world. They ate fruit for breakfast and that was all. Undressed salad and nuts for lunch. More salad—lots of sprouts!—and maybe a baked potato for dinner. If they were going all out, they'd put some avocado on the potato. I don't know about you, but when I think of the culinary good life, that isn't it.

It would be years later, when clever raw chefs began to create actual cuisine from uncooked fruits, vegetables, nuts, and seeds, that I seriously looked at "raw" as something that might be for me. I soon realized that for many people, myself included, an *all*-raw diet, even a delicious one, can be too restrictive. And other than for a short cleanse, the whole thing can seem bizarre, with the wheatgrass and Himalayan berries and recipes that begin: "Break a young Thai coconut with your machete." Besides, from November to May, raw is just plain cold. As a result, lots of folks dabble in it, but most of them give it up. I'm here to rescue the dabblers and suggest that you eat a veritable cornucopia of uncooked vegetables and fruits, especially in warm weather, and the very best cooked foods, too. It's about color *and* comfort, about living foods *and* living life.

To eat raw in cold weather, bring refrigerated foods to room temperature before eating; heat soups to under 118°F on the stove or in a high-powered blender; use warming spices such as ginger, curry, and chiles; when you come inside, warm up by the fireplace or with a hot bath or cup of tea before you have your meal; and wear warm clothing, layers, and even those toe-warmers made for skiers.

The sweet spot for well-being comes from finding the ideal balance of bright, brilliant foods just as they come from the orchard and garden, while allowing for cooked foods, as well, with their variety, leeway in social situations, warmth in the winter, and some comforting nutrient insurance.

Beans and whole grains are rich in certain minerals, amino acids, and B vitamins that can be tricky to get with all raw food; and a few phytonutrients—the lycopene in tomatoes, for instance—are actually more accessible when you eat the food cooked. Grounding cooked dishes provide staying power and needed calories that fruits and vegetables don't always have, and that you don't want to get from an excess of high-fat foods—nuts, seeds, avocado—even though these are highly beneficial in moderation.

An appreciation of raw foods, but without taking any vows or signing any pledges, qualifies a person as a "raw enthusiast." That's the category into which I put myself and to which I extend you a cordial invitation. It's easy to be enthusiastic about raw foods because eating them gives you a huge vitality boost. And once you recover from the "palate perversion" most of us developed from eating greasy foods and too-sweet sweets, the flavor burst from a perfect peach or a savory salad can be borderline orgasmic.

Even so, during the cold seasons (in New York we have two-and-a-half cold seasons), I need more warm, cooked-for-comfort meals. Besides, William (my husband) might leave me if I didn't make veggie chili once a week through the winter. I'm fond of having a baby-it's-cold-outside pot of soup on hand; and my standby lunch, when a giant salad just won't cut it, is "Beans 'n' Greens." To make this, I sauté onions, garlic (I like elephant garlic: giant cloves that peel and chop easily), mushrooms, and red beans or black beans or chickpeas. Then I add something vibrantly green—broccoli or baby kale or spinach or arugula—and sauté just a bit longer. (A note here, and a confession, I suppose: I buy canned beans, as long as the label says those cans are free of the endocrine-disrupting chemical BPA. Eden Organic, Westbrae Natural, Trader Joe's, and Native Forest have phased out BPA in either all or some of their cans.)

If I'll be out at lunchtime, I might stop at a Chinese restaurant for steamed veggies with tofu and brown rice, black bean sauce on the side; or at a soup-and-salad place where I can get hot (vegan) soup and some raw veggies, too. On chilly mornings I often make an "oatmeal parfait," a veritable cereal still life with fresh fruits and berries, ground flaxseeds, chopped walnuts, and a delicate drizzle of maple syrup. If I make a smoothie instead, I skip the ice or frozen fruit. And I have tea every morning. Sometimes it's antioxidant-rich green tea or a caffeine-free spiced chai, but my favorite is fragrant Earl Grey with frothy almond milk, an affection I developed when I lived in London fresh out of high school, figuring out who I was going to be.

GKT

Spices can be powerful antioxidants. Cloves top the list, along with turmeric, ginger, cayenne, oregano, garlic, and cinnamon. Look for Ceylon cinnamon; the more common variety contains a potentially carcinogenic compound.

Despite the role cooked selections can play in a healthy diet, raw food is healthy eating turbocharged. Fresh, raw vegetables, fruits, and sprouts have their life force fully intact. Plant a raw carrot and you'll get a carrot; plant a cooked carrot and you'll get compost. It's fine to eat a cooked carrot (or any other whole, plant food); just know that the more cooked it is, the more liveliness it's lost. That's certainly one reason why, when it's warm outside and I'm feeling my very best, I'm consuming mostly:

- Fresh juices—greens and lemon are my go-to, but I'm also getting into blends that include beet juice, shown to enhance athletic performance

- Gardens of greens—in salads, marinated, or tossed into smoothies

- Other vegetables, including sea vegetables and some fermented veggies (kimchi and sauerkraut)

- Sprouts grown on my kitchen counter

- Fruit, organic when I can get it, or from a nearly organic area orchard when I can't

- Nuts and seeds, occasionally munched but usually made into a yummy dressing or dip, a pâté, nut milk, or a luxurious dessert

- And sometimes a raw delicacy from the health food store— an exquisite nut cheese (I'm a great fan of both Treeline and Miyoko's Kitchen cheeses), crackers (flaxseed mostly, dehydrated at low heat), and raw granola, made from coconut or buckwheat, also dehydrated. (People who get very excited about raw cuisine often purchase a dehydrator and make these treats themselves. I'm not that domestic, and your closet is probably bigger than my kitchen, so I don't have a dehydrator.)

I will use salad dressing with some flax or hemp or (most often) olive oil in it. Some people don't believe in using any oil, and it is a fact that the studies showing reversal of even severe cardiovascular disease had subjects on an oil-free diet. As of today, I feel balanced and nourished and lean doing what I'm doing. If that stops working for me, I'll do something different.

I avoid refined sugar almost entirely, but I'm not afraid of fruit. Berries, in particular, are veritable antioxidant bunkers, and an apple spread with nut butter makes a yummy quick lunch with romaine leaves and celery. I put bananas in smoothies; I love peaches and persimmons and pineapple; and I make desserts with dates—a whole food—or a little pure maple syrup or coconut sugar.

Coconut sugar is the latest super-sweetener, said to be low on the glycemic index and an altogether wonderful thing. Of course, that used to be the hype about agave nectar, now maligned as little better than high-fructose corn syrup. The heart of the matter is that sweeteners, of whatever origin, are sweet. They're treats, not entitlements. And when life is really sweet, you don't need nearly as much dessert.

Marissa's Good Karma Story

When I was a child, I'd give up small things for Lent—like quarreling with my little brother. On the eve of Lent fifteen years ago, I decided to do something truly meaningful, to make what seemed like a real sacrifice in order to make a difference: I gave up meat. I don't remember if I initially had the intention to stay meat-free after Lent or not, but I knew my fate was sealed after one particular cafeteria lunch. I ate a bite of my friend's chicken nugget, a momentary lapse in my vow, and was immediately flooded with sadness and disgust. I couldn't stop thinking about that chicken—not the inanimate object on the tray, but the formerly living, breathing, feeling, and suffering chicken that I had consumed. Once I made that connection, there was no turning back. In a few short years, I was full-on vegan.

My veganism, rooted in animal liberation, was a gateway to my passion for environmentalism, human rights, and healthy living. I began to really take care of myself and extend that care to those around me. Then, ten years after my life-changing decision, disaster struck. Literally overnight, I went from healthy and athletic to dangerously ill and bedridden, every night fearing I'd not live to see the next day. I eventually found out that toxic mold had robbed me of my healthy life. Since I was in bed for months, I had a lot of time to analyze my condition. My doctors continually told me to eat eggs and fish to strengthen and rebalance my system, but with my knowledge of vegan nutrition, I refused.

When I was well enough to begin caring for myself again, I first adopted an unprocessed, high-raw, vegan diet (in contrast to my previous diet, which was higher in heavily processed vegan foods). Then I bought a juicer and began to use it. Instantly, my health began to improve. I also started to realize that because I'd eaten relatively well and taken care of my body for so many years, I was strong enough to fight off this crazy illness. Veganism literally saved my life.

As I reflect on my journey, I realize that karma is a cyclical pattern that continues on. I gave something—something I first thought of as a sacrifice but later regarded as a compassionate choice—and years later I was given something in return: my health.

But it doesn't stop there. Because of the gift I was given, I have a strong urge in my life to give back. In other words, health was not the only gift that veganism gave me; I realized my life's purpose as well. At some point, I stopped living my life only for my recovery and started living it so that I'd be better able to help others overcome their unique health challenges, too. I feel pure joy when helping others live more vibrantly, and I want to do it to the best of my ability. I wanted to educate myself, and I began that process by getting certified as a Vegan Lifestyle Coach and Educator through Main Street Vegan Academy. And so the karmic cycle continues.

—**Marissa Podany**, VLCE (Vegan Lifestyle Coach and Educator), blogger. RevelinginRaw.blogspot.com

5

......

High-Green, High-Raw, High-Energy Eating

The how-to is simple: Eat food that is beautiful and delicious, and eat enough of it. Most raw, plant food is very low in calories and it is possible to get too thin. Besides, being hungry is unnecessary and distracting: who wants to be vexed by a gurgling tummy when you've got a life to live?

There's also too much delicious, healthful, rejuvenating food out there for you to eat anything you don't enjoy. Refuse to force any substance down your gullet that you're not pleased to be consuming. (Have I mentioned that I don't do wheatgrass shots? They make me gag. Life's too short.) True, some of the stronger greens and stranger fruits are acquired tastes. Give yourself a chance to acquire them, but if you're not feeling the love, move on. People who try to keep track of such things report that there are between four hundred and nine hundred cultivated vegetables, and sometimes thousands of varieties of a single one. You won't run out.

For breakfast, know thyself. Honor your personal proclivities. Some people wake up ravenous and others need to be up awhile before food sounds good—but do eat something in the morning. The studies on centenarians cite that, however else these folks differ, and they differ a lot, they're invariably breakfast-eaters. For your long-life breakfast, choose one or two dishes from the following:

- *Fresh juice* with greens in it—romaine/kale/apple/lemon; tomato/arugula/lemon; cucumber/collards/celery/pear; spinach/cucumber/celery/pineapple

- *Fruit and nuts*—have an ounce or two of walnuts or macadamias, or your favorite raw nut butter, or a nut or seed cheese, with romaine leaves and celery and fruits in season (include berries, low in sugar and rich in antioxidants, as often as you can).

- *Fruit smoothie* with a nondairy milk or nondairy yogurt base. If you like, add a vegan protein powder—those made from Brazil nut or hemp protein are often raw—and some "superfood" addition that makes you feel super-powered. Among these are Ceylon cinnamon (terrific antioxidant), maca (an adaptogen said to enhance energy and help regulate hormones), or ground flaxseeds (they contain ALA, an omega-3 fatty acid, and lignans shown to protect against breast cancer).

- *Green smoothie*—my favorite green smoothie is unsweetened coconut milk, spinach, pineapple, and either a frozen banana (for a thicker piña colada smoothie) or just ice cubes for a light, refreshing cooler.

- *Raw cereal* (raw granola, muesli, soaked chia seeds) with fresh nut milk or other nondairy milk, ground flaxseeds, fresh fruit and berries

- *Hot cereal*, such as oatmeal, millet, or quinoa, with fresh and dried fruits and berries, ground flaxseeds, chopped walnuts, and maybe a teeny sprinkle of ground clove—this spice has the highest antioxidant content of any food in common usage.

- *Sprouted grain, "sun-fired" bread*, with nut butter, apple, or banana. The breads I'm referring to come in little mound-shaped loaves; one brand is "Manna Bread." These aren't raw—that would require heating under 118°F, the temperature at which the enzymes present in natural foods are killed—but they're baked at lower heat than conventional breads, minimizing the potential for creating the carcinogenic acrylamide that occurs during regular baking and other high-heat cooking processes.

One of these "other processes" is the roasting of coffee beans. In California, where the government is interested in protecting its citizens from potential carcinogens, an acrylamide notice is posted in coffee shops, noting that this plastic-like substance forms as a result of high heat and applies, in these restaurants, to both the coffee and the baked goods. There are cold-processed coffees at some natural foods stores and restaurants, if you wish to seek these out. Obviously, some people don't do well with the caffeine in coffee, either, and women prone to fibrocystic breast changes are advised to stay away from it. Still, studies have found benefits to its consumption, too, notably a decreased incidence of dementia in elderly people consuming a substantial amount of the stuff, four or more cups a day.

My own plan is to protect my brain with exercise and blueberries, and avoid that cuppa joe except for medicinal purposes (e.g., jet lag). I do get caffeine in the morning in my tea (black has more than green; both have less than coffee; and you can modulate the amount with the steeping time). Should you wish to go cold-tofu on caffeine, realize that there's the potential for headaches, shakes, and irritability.

Easing off—coffee to black tea to green tea to caffeine-free beverages—works best. And if you love the aroma, the richness, and the ritual of coffee, Teeccino (www.teeccino.com) is an herbal wonder you brew in your coffeemaker—all the pleasure, none of the caffeine. Another tip: If you crave caffeine in the mid-afternoon, try a fresh green juice instead. It has remarkable pick-me-up potential.

For lunch, start with a colorful vegetable juice, if available, then select:

- *A giant salad.* Add *oomph* factor—that's what keeps this from being "just a salad"—with steamed broccoli or asparagus; cubes of steamed sweet potato or squash; cooked quinoa or barley; beans (small red beans are super high in antioxidants, or choose kidney beans, black beans, lentils, chickpeas—they're all good); and toss with a nut-based dressing or lemon and avocado. If you're especially hungry, have some raw flax crackers or whole-grain bread with hummus or seed pâté. (Leftovers of last night's cooked entrée can also give some extra staying power to your lunchtime salad.)

- *Soup*—a raw blended soup based on tomatoes or greens, or a cooked bean or vegetable soup, with raw veggies (with or without dip), and flax crackers or bread and spread as above

- *A wrap*, using collard or romaine leaves or your favorite whole-grain flatbread as the wrapper, with a nut, seed, or bean pâté or spread, raw veggies—think of this as a handheld salad—fruit for dessert

- *Sushi!* Make nori wraps with seed pâté or sticky short-grain brown rice with avocado or cucumber, and serve with miso soup and edamame.

- *A sliced apple* spread with nut butter, celery sticks, romaine leaves, a couple of Medjool dates, and maybe some of that Manna bread

- *Any of the breakfast options* that bear repeating

GKT

Seasoned rice vinegar is a remarkable product that tastes rich, almost oily, and can dress a salad all on its own. If you don't see it with the other vinegars in your supermarket, look in the Asian section.

For **dinner**, have your second glass of fresh juice (or your first, if you haven't enjoyed that yet), and then choose any items from the breakfast or luncheon listings, or:

- *Caesar salad* with sea vegetables—dulse is lovely—and finely grated nondairy cheese

- *Gourmet raw entrée*—lasagna or pasta marinara using sliced or spiralized zucchini or commercially available kelp noodles—with a salad

- *Rib-sticking cooked vegan entrée*—beans, tempeh, black or brown or red rice, quinoa, and whole-grain pasta all work as main dish bases. Accompany your entrée with one or more steamed vegetables (broccoli, asparagus, string beans, carrots, kale), and a good-sized salad.

- *Beans and greens*—I gave you basic instructions in chapter 4, and Doris has provided a fancier, Thai-inspired recipe,

Thai Greens and Beans, in Appendix A (see page 259). Serve with a raw side dish, perhaps a Caprese salad: tomatoes, nut cheese, and fresh basil—again, there's a recipe, Cheesy Caprese, in Appendix A (see page 249).

- A *steamed sweet potato* topped with avocado and ground Himalayan salt (this is unrefined salt with its mineral content intact), *or baked winter squash*, drizzled with flaxseed oil and pure maple syrup and topped with walnut halves. Accompany with a sizable green salad sprinkled with hemp seeds, and a steamed vegetable—asparagus, broccoli, cauliflower, spinach, string beans, zucchini.

- *Tex-Mex bar*—Kids and company love a big salad of romaine and leaf lettuce, with south-of-the-border additions: guacamole, salsa, beans or refried beans (a total misnomer—they've never been fried), sautéed onions and peppers, shredded nondairy cheese, and baked organic corn chips or Mexican-flavored raw flax crackers.

Should you want a sweet, look to fruit as the dessert of first resort: I often serve orange slices, like some Chinese restaurants do. Otherwise, consider a raw treat, made from real food. These desserts are full-flavored and delicious—you won't need much. (Let Doris tempt you with her recipes in Appendix A.) A little piece of high-cacao-content dark chocolate is a simple, low-sugar way to sweetly end a meal, and so are a couple tablespoons of nuts in a custard cup. We've all heard the phrase "from soup to nuts." I don't know why ending a meal with creamy hazelnuts, pecans, or macadamias (these have an excellent omega-3-to-omega-6 ratio) doesn't happen more often. The richness of nuts makes them dessert-like with no sugar at all.

If you're used to having wine with dinner, one glass for a woman, two for a man, is said to be moderate, and modest consumption of red wine is routinely recommended as a way to lower cholesterol. Some studies suggest that, at the one- to two-drink-per-day level, *any* alcohol intake correlates with longer life. On the other hand, there is concern that alcohol, even in small amounts, may be a factor in the development of breast cancer. That's enough of a concern to me that I generally avoid wine and spirits. But you know what? I never really liked to drink. It always made me sleepy instead of sociable, so not indulging is no big deal for me. If you enjoy a glass of wine, that enjoyment is worth something. Read up on the pros and cons and determine that whatever you decide about imbibing, you'll always feel just right about it.

Dee's Good Karma Story

I never consciously set out be a vegan and certainly never even dreamed of adopting a raw lifestyle. I have come to believe that I did not choose these paths: they chose me. My consciousness of animal suffering and my growing awareness of nutrition have been the catalysts for a new life. Not only am I happier and healthier than I have ever been, but I also successfully started my own business to share what I've discovered.

I grew up in an average meat-and-potatoes family. My dad was a recreational hunter and an avid fisherman. My earliest memories are of trolling for bluefish in the waters of Cape Cod, and spearing eels in salt marshes at night. Growing up in Boston in the 1960s and '70s, I didn't know anyone who was vegetarian, and when I heard the word, I had the vision of an emaciated, sprout-munching radical. I wrote off vegetarians as members of a fringe group, to be tolerated at best and, preferably, avoided.

Fast-forward to 1981 and college. I finally met a real live vegetarian: my assigned roommate. I genuinely liked her and her veg friends, so I decided to shun meat, too. Ironically, it was a desire to fit in with a group that didn't really fit in that uncovered my authentic nature.

I continued my vegetarian diet for some thirty years and thought I was doing okay, despite periods of low energy, depression, inflammation, and headaches, as well as skin and digestive disturbances. I assumed this was a normal part of the aging process, and it was not the impetus for my shift to veganism. That came from learning about the realities of factory farming. In my mind, dairy cows had always been happy creatures in green pastures, just beyond where chickens roamed freely in big barnyards. Once I released my delusion that the most disturbing form of animal cruelty was raising livestock for beef, my transition was easy: the next morning, I woke up vegan.

On the surface, my progression to a raw lifestyle was also unexpected, but I believe it was an intentional part of some divine plan for me. I came to see that plant-based food, fresh from the earth, is powerful, energetic, healthy, sacred, medicinal, artistic, simple, nourishing, and revolutionary. It's peace and love for all. This is my food philosophy. Today, at age fifty-two, I am a very healthy individual in body, mind, and spirit. I'm happy and have a positive attitude. Physical discomforts are rare. My skin glows and I have boundless energy. I quite literally walked away from a toxic job and dove into my intended life's purpose without any thought of a safety net. It turned out to be one of the best decisions I ever made.

I am the proud owner of my own company that creates and markets raw, vegan, and organic "sun sweets and savories." My foods are crafted with compassion and my ideas are inspired by sunshine, an approach I like to apply to all my life's endeavors. It is my hope and my intention to create a positive change in our world simply by sharing sun food with others, as well as promoting a plant-based lifestyle through personal experience and example. May there be peace on earth for all living and sentient beings.

—**Dee Edwards**, owner and creator of dee's good food.
DeesGoodFood.com

6

......

21 Days to Good Health and Good Karma

'm not always a fan of "doing a detox"—going all the way and then some for a prescribed amount of time. It can make you feel incredibly fit and beautiful and accomplished, but if it feels at all restrictive—the "and then some" often does—it's human nature to rebel, to return with a vengeance to old comforts and old patterns.

Nevertheless, far too many people to overlook have told me that this process—a juice cleanse, or a period on all raw food, or a couple of weeks in the boot camp atmosphere of a natural healing center or spa—initiated their lasting, healthy, vegan lifestyle. To this end, then, I offer you an optional 21-day plan to change some routines, detox from animal foods and processed foods, and give you a head start on the changes you'll be making anyhow. I strongly advise that you do this as preparation for a new way of relating to food and your body, rather than as a parenthesis inserted into your life, with status quo habits on either side.

Here's the plan: For the next 21 days, you're going to follow nine simple instructions. I like nine. In feng shui, it's the number of completion, and if you opt to do this, I want you to *complete* the 21-day program and extract from it every possible morsel of well-being, vitality, and inspiration. If you slip, just get up and keep going. Since this is a detox program, it's more regimented than your Good Karma Life afterward needs to be, but these three weeks will give you a sense of what really clean living feels like. If afterward you want to go back to coffee, or include some processed foods, or return to a late-night schedule, that's your business. The foundational Good Karma aspects of your future choices—quality food, no animals—will, ideally, be with you for keeps.

You will need to devote some time to this each day, so schedule your foray into body bliss accordingly—maybe beginning your detox on a weekend or, even better, when you have a few days off. Note that each suggestion also includes an additional action, "extra karmic credit." Do all, some, or none of the extra-credit options. This isn't about overachieving; it's about blossoming.

GKT

Stay hydrated by consuming filtered water and water-rich raw fruits and veggies, fresh juices, and herbal teas. Ayurveda recommends sipping throughout the day warm water with a touch of lemon or essential oil of lemon (the Young Living oils are edible). How much water do you need? Turn your weight into ounces, cut it in half, and drink that much, e.g., a 140-pound person needs 70 ounces of water each day.

The instructions are:

1. Comprise your diet solely of vegetables, greens, and sprouts; fresh fruits; legumes; raw nuts and seeds; and

gluten-free whole grains (skip the wheat, rye, barley, farro, and spelt). For now, don't eat anything else—nothing from a factory (make your own nut milk even—Doris has given you a recipe, Brazil Nut Milk, in Appendix A on page 228) and no alcohol. Ideally, soak any nuts you eat or use in a recipe (unless the recipe specifies unsoaked nuts) in water for a few hours or up to overnight to facilitate digestion. *Extra karmic credit: Switch from coffee and black tea to lower-caffeine green tea or, if you're feeling like a mighty warrior, scale back over these 21 days to herbal coffees and teas with no caffeine at all.*

2. **Depending on the season and how you do with raw food, strive to make 75 percent (or more) of your food intake uncooked.** *Extra karmic credit: Have a 16-ounce glass of fresh, green juice daily. Focus on celery, cucumber, and romaine lettuce, all of which make a lot of juice, plus spinach, kale, broccoli stems (juicing loves leftovers), parsley, collard greens, and Swiss chard—less juice, more potency. Always include lemon (peeled) so your green juice won't taste grassy, and a little apple or pear for sweetness, but keep those to a minimum since fruit juice, when separated from its fibrous casing, becomes an "unprotected simple sugar," best consumed only in small amounts.*

3. **Have a least one giant salad each day.** Serve it with a nut-based dressing, or avocado and lemon. *Extra karmic credit: Rotate your leafies—Bibb lettuce, leaf lettuce, romaine lettuce, arugula, frisée, mizuna, mesclun greens, spinach, Swiss chard, bok choy, cabbage, radicchio, and massaged kale or collards. To do the massaging, drizzle with some olive oil, lemon juice, or apple cider vinegar, and good-quality salt; then rub and knead and squeeze the greens with your hands to tenderize them. If you then let your greens rest for an hour or*

so, they'll be as tender as if they were cooked. Use other produce—red bell pepper, black olives, shredded carrots, dried cranberries—to add bright spots of color and additional nutrition to any salad.

GKT

Dress up your salad with artichoke hearts, sugar snap peas, water chestnuts, dried cherries or blueberries, mandarin orange sections, even vegan bacon-y bits—my pick for those is Frontier Organic Bac'uns from VeganEssentials.com.

4. **Go to bed by 10 p.m. and get up by 6 a.m.—6:30 at the latest.** According to Ayurveda, that ancient Indian philosophy still recognized by the World Health Organization as a legitimate health care system, sleeping and waking on this schedule puts you in tune with nature's cycles and allows your body to function best. I've also observed that most of the people who make a real difference on this planet are early risers. *Extra karmic credit: Turn off the TV, computer, and other electronic devices one hour before bedtime. Spend that time reading, doing some gentle yoga, or cozying up with your true love. And while you're at it, charge those electronics somewhere other than your bedroom to protect yourself from exposure to electromagnetic field radiation.*

5. Meditate—sit, watch your breath, or mentally say a mantra, a calming word or phrase—for at least ten minutes, preferably twenty, every morning. Alternatively, use this as time for prayer, scripture reading, journal

writing—whatever appeals to you and could be described as "meditative." *Extra karmic credit: Do this again later in the day—after work but before dinner is recommended; before bed works, too. The majority of the scientific studies showing the positive effects of meditation on health have looked at people using the Transcendental Meditation technique, a mantra meditation, twenty minutes twice a day. (For more how and why on meditation, treat yourself to* Success Through Stillness, *by Russell Simmons—the hip-hop mogul and yogi who is also a vegan.)*

6. Do formal exercise six days a week. Choose from activities you enjoy—yoga class, Pilates, biking, rock climbing, roller skating, parkour—so long as you're including:
   - cardiovascular exercise (i.e., you sweat but can still have a conversation) for at least thirty minutes a minimum of four times a week.

   - full-body strength training at least twice a week (you can divide this up and do two days upper body, two days lower body, with a full day off between body parts; work your core every time).

   - stretching after your workouts, plus some gentle bedtime and wakeup stretches, just like your dog or cat does.

   Extra karmic credit: Bring the cardio up to forty-five minutes. Even the treadmill isn't tedious if you're watching a movie or listening to a podcast while you do it.

7. Boost your body's detox efforts by adopting at least two of the following practices during the 21 days:
   - *Clean your tongue* with an inexpensive tongue scraper from your pharmacy or natural food store. Every morning, gently scrape off the buildup that collects there during

the night. In Ayurveda, this is called *ama*, "metabolic debris" that you want to be rid of. At the very least, it's great for freshening your breath for real, rather than relying on a minty cover-up.

- *Try oil pulling.* No worries if you avoid oil in your diet: this is rinsing your mouth with oil, not consuming it. Sesame oil is used most often, or coconut or almond oil. Take a tablespoon or so in your mouth and swish it around somewhat vigorously for about fifteen minutes. I sometimes do this in the morning while I check my e-mail. When you're finished, spit the oil into a plastic-lined trash can. This process apparently has a detergent-like ability to clear the mouth and gums of bacteria, and many people who practice oil pulling report whiter teeth and an improvement in periodontal health. (If you want to know more, look up *Oil-Pulling Therapy,* by Dr. Bruce Fife.)

- *Learn to use a neti pot.* Once the purview only of yogis (adventurous ones, at that), the neti pot for nasal cleansing is now sold in drugstores, recommended by ENT specialists, and showcased on *Dr. Oz.* The pot looks like a little Aladdin's lamp, and it will come with detailed instructions. Basically, you'll fill it with warm water and ⅛ to ¼ teaspoon finely ground salt (the kind sold specifically for this use is ideal, but noniodized table salt will work). Bend over a sink far enough that your nose is parallel to the floor, allowing the saline solution to cleanse one sinus passage and come out the opposite nostril. Don't inhale! Then do the other side. This can be especially useful if you suffer from allergies or are prone to colds. (For additional information, see *The Neti Pot for Better Health,* by Warren Jefferson.)

- *Perform deep-breathing exercises.* If you do yoga regularly, you're already a breathing pro. The rest of us need to remind ourselves to get in some serious inhalations and exhalations—at least ten in the morning and ten at night, ideally outside or near an open window. (If there's a "halotherapy" place near you, experience an hour in a "salt cave." It's purported to benefit lung function and is, at the very least, deeply relaxing.)

- *Do dry skin brushing.* Purchase a dry skin brush at the health food store or a nice drugstore (be sure it's made of plant fibers—no boar bristles) and before your bath or shower, brush your body. Start with your feet and move up, using long strokes along the long bones and round, gentle moves over your abdomen and chest. Skip your face—these bristles are too tough for that tender skin. Dry skin brushing will help reduce the amount of dead skin cells that are keeping you from glowing and that impede the ability of your skin, your largest organ by area, from optimally performing its detoxification tasks.

- *Got sweat?* I know you're sweating with your aerobic exercise, but sweating in a sauna—a "far infrared" sauna, if you have access to one—may be a worthy addition. A far infrared sauna is said to heat you from the inside (I know, it all sounds rather alternative . . .) and some legit studies from Europe suggest that repeated periods of sweating in this way can reduce the load of heavy metals many of us carry from eating, drinking, and breathing at this time in history. You can actually purchase a fold-up, one-person sauna for about $250. Mine gets the most use in the winter when I come in from braving the elements.

- *Take a probiotic capsule every morning before breakfast.* We can get so used to our bodies' functioning in a certain way that it seems normal, even if it's not. Digestion is like that. Unless we're having a stomachache or noticeable bloating or constipation, everything seems okay. See what happens to "okay" with the assistance of a nondairy probiotic boost once a day. Most people love how they feel with this addition of friendly bacteria to their digestive apparatus. Taking a probiotic, ideally a combination of acidophilus and bifidus strains, also helps your system get used to eating more raw foods and high-fiber foods—healthful, to be sure, but something new for your body to deal with. Any discomfort you might experience in changing to this type of diet is somewhat like the soreness that comes with starting to exercise: it's a transitory thing. Go slowly if you need to. If your diet has been fairly typical, relying on animal foods, refined carbs, or both, know that juices, smoothies, blended salads, and fermented foods can be easier to digest than lots of beans, raw vegetables, and nuts right off the bat. Taking a probiotic may ease the transition.

- *Indulge in a professional massage if you can.* Ideally, try some bodywork you've never had before—maybe Thai yoga massage (lots of passive stretching), shiatsu (pressure point work to release deep tension), or manual lymphatic drainage (MLD), a gentle technique designed to assist your lymphatic system, the body's premier detoxifier, in getting its job done.

Extra karmic credit: Try all of the above and adopt a few as lifelong habits.

8. **Keep a log of your experience.** If you're a journal-keeper, include it there. If not, make an account, electronically or on

paper, of what you're eating, what you're doing, how you're feeling, and what clever ideas come into your joyfully detoxed brain during this experience. *Extra karmic credit: Share your log, and your process, with a detox buddy. Take this 21-day at-home journey in the company of a friend, talking and e-mailing daily.*

After your detox, continue with plant-based eating and whatever other practices you believe are enriching your life. A great diet, regular exercise, meditation, and adequate sleep on a regular schedule are the fundamentals for feeling really well every day and laying the foundation for lifelong health. Find a way to make these practices part of your routine. You did even more for three whole weeks. Going forward, it's just a day at a time.

7

......

Good Cheer and a
Good Blender

You don't need a lot of equipment or gadgets to be a Good Karma cook—an unfortunate term, perhaps, when we're talking about eating more raw food, but you get my gist. Nevertheless, you do want a kitchen outfitted for the preparation of food. Whether you're a full-fledged, high-raw vegan, or for now just adding more produce to your culinary repertoire, you'll be healthier—and, I believe, more centered, too—if you prepare most meals at home and depend less on cafés and carry-out. This way you'll know what's in everything, and your food won't be laced with iffy chemicals because that's just not something you'd do. Preparing food at home will also save you money so when you do dine out, you can choose to go someplace dazzling.

GKT

Rethink fast food: On a Good Karma Diet, fast food is fruit. Berries: rinse and eat. Banana: peel and eat. Cantaloupe: halve, seed, and eat.

Here's my short (and cheap) list of equipment that should make your preparation of natural, plant foods easy and fun:

- **Knives.** A chef's knife (big one) and a paring knife, plus a sharpener you've learned how to use, make a worthy start.

- **Cutting board.** I like Lucite since it can go in the dishwasher, but wood is lovely if you're willing to care for it with gentle hand-washing and periodic oiling.

- **Bowls.** Start with large salad bowls, sometimes called pasta bowls, for yourself and family members who'll be joining in, even if only part of the time. You'll also need a huge salad bowl—I get mine at a restaurant supply house—for tossing greens and other additions.

- **Steaming trivet.** This inexpensive gadget—ten bucks or under—goes inside a pot with some boiling water so you can steam veggies without their touching the water and losing valuable nutrients. Because a variety of plant foods cooked at very high heat can develop acrylamide, that plastic-like coating believed to be carcinogenic, I've given up baking even starchy vegetables such as sweet potatoes and butternut squash. They taste delicious steamed and the prep time is only a third that of baking. (A bamboo steamer—see "Diana's Good Karma Story" at the end of this chapter—is another way to go.)

- **Blender.** Choose either a good-quality standard blender (Oster makes fine ones; so do Breville and Cuisinart), or a high-powered blender, such as the Vitamix or Blendtec. These cost quite a bit more but do more, too. I finally got a Vitamix a couple of years ago (thanks, Santa); it saves me time and my green smoothies are decidedly smoother than the ones I made before. Is it a necessity? No—it's like a sports car: not required for getting to work, but a really nice ride.

Some other items you'll want to add as soon as you can are a :

- **Food processor.** If you don't have one now, you can get by with only a blender for the time being, but blenders are at their best whizzing up smoothies, soups, dressings, and sauces, while a food processor is designed to make short work of thicker concoctions, such as a spread, pâté, or raw cake batter, piecrust, or other confections based on nuts and dried fruit. Your food processor can also chop and shred in short order.

- **Juicer,** one capable of extracting juice from greens, as well as from carrots, celery, cucumbers, and fruits. Unless you plan to purchase fresh juice daily from a juice bar, you need to be able to make it yourself. I juice in the late afternoon. It's a ritual. I juice, then meditate. I'd like to have dinner at six, but William often works later; juice and meditation tide me over. Having owned several juicers over the years, I've had my share of disappointments. My current juicer, the Breville Juice Fountain, works well for me. It's small enough for my kitchen, easy to clean (that's important), and juices greens, not bone-dry like some pricey juicers that resemble army tanks, but quite well, thank you.

- **Spiralizer.** This makes spaghetti-like strands and spirals from zucchini, sweet potato, and a few other vegetables. It's manual and a quite serviceable one can be had for under $40.

- **Citrus juicer.** Choose manual or electric: with this type of food prep, you'll be using quite a bit of lemon juice.

- Coffee grinder or nut mill—Use this small (mine was $10) device to grind your flaxseeds and, if you're a foodie through and through, to grind fresh spices.

With this equipment, or most of it, you can prepare delicious food with minimal fuss. If adventurous dining isn't high on your list of earthly pleasures, you'll do beautifully with basic meals. Put together in some appealing way foods the sun has already cooked and, if you like, add something a bit more complex (if steamed broccoli counts as complex). Other than a knife, I don't think William has ever used one of the pieces of equipment listed, and yet on the nights when I'm out or otherwise not making dinner, he does quite well for himself. A typical guy-night meal for him is a salad of leafy greens and tomato with avocado, canned beans, and maybe a couple of ears of sweet corn when it's in season—blanched in boiling water, or even raw if it's fresh and sweet from the farmers' market.

At the height of summer, he may eat peaches, plums, and nectarines, with romaine lettuce leaves and celery, and have a glass or two of soy or almond milk before bed. When winter sets in and fresh foods aren't as abundant or attractive, he'll accompany a smaller salad with some veggie-meat, or a couple of vegan tuna salad sandwiches (the spread might be store-bought, or one I've whipped up from tofu, chickpeas, or sunflower seeds—it's the spices that make it reminiscent of a familiar food from the past). And there's always the inner-child standby, PB&J (peanuts-only peanut butter, of course, and all-fruit jam).

You, on the other hand, unlike my husband, may love working with food. If you find it relaxing and creative and the kitchen feels like your mother ship, you'll have fun with recipe books and Googling whatever seems impossible. Look for raw mashed potatoes, maybe (quite possible, but the "potatoes" are cauliflower, as in Doris's Masquerading Mashed "Potatoes" recipe in Appendix A on page 265); or raw, vegan fudge (cacao powder, dates, nut butter—this one's a piece of cake).

One larger appliance that people who are serious about raw cuisine usually acquire at some point is a dehydrator. When foods are heated at low heat (maxing out at somewhere between 110 and 118°F, depending whom you ask), their enzymatic activity remains intact and they're still considered raw. With a dehydrator, you can stay within these guidelines and make raw crackers, cookies, loaves, hard cheeses, and unleavened breads, as well as dried fruits and fruit leather, vegetable chips, and crispy soaked nuts. (Soaking deactivates the enzyme inhibitors in nuts and makes them more digestible, but once soaked, you need to keep them refrigerated and eat them within five days. Dehydrating increases their "shelf life" and provides a welcome crunch, almost like roasting.)

As I said back in chapter 4, I don't own a dehydrator due to lack of space, and I'm not sure I'd get one anyway. Because the process can take many hours, dehydrating calls for a complete rethink on food prep. Since what I prize most about raw foods is their juiciness, their high water content, I'm not eager to remove that moisture to make a cracker. Perhaps if I aspired to be "all raw," I'd purchase a dehydrator, even if I had to keep it in the living room, but since I have no problem using my stove, I'm one appliance closer to the joys of the simple life.

Diana's Good Karma Story

My evolution toward a plant-based diet gave me this sweet and surprising gift: the creative joy of cooking without a recipe. I discovered my inner cooking artist. It was like going from coloring within the lines to painting freely at an easel. I could now choose from a multitude of grains and multicolored vegetables, decide on an appealing spice or ethnic flavor, and select a Good Karma, earth-friendly source of concentrated protein.

Now when I stand in the kitchen, I scan my cupboards and refrigerator the way a collage artist gathers the pieces with which she has to work. I cook dinner in short order and, even after a long day at the office, find creative contentment in the process. Cooking with vegetables peacefully grounds me.

It all starts with the shopping trip—my kind of shopping. Given a choice between Whole Foods and Nordstrom's, it's Whole Foods for me, hands down. Today's shopping list has over fifteen fruits and vegetables. The colors, textures, flavors, and nutrients figuratively and literally feed me.

My favorite way of preparing vegetables is to steam them in a ten-inch bamboo steamer, the type you see in a packed-to-the-brim Japanese store (or on Amazon). I layer the vegetables according to their needed cooking times. The firmer vegetables comprise the bottom layer; the more delicate beauties are on top. Bamboo steaming allows for the best flavor, color, and texture. My assortment always includes some red cabbage, broccoli, cauliflower, carrots, beets, and sturdy kale. I sometimes add chunks of squash, sweet potato, eggplant, or some other vegetable that caught my eye in the store.

I follow the steaming with an ice bath to retain a bright color and an al dente texture. The process doesn't take long, and it pays off with both a quick dinner and a week's worth of vegetables for lunches. I make this a pleasant experience, usually on Sunday morning during the only TV show I watch regularly, *Sunday Morning*. As the vegetables are steaming, I make a sauce—maybe garlic tahini or my favorite: romesco sauce, a Spanish delicacy based on nuts and roasted red peppers. The finishing touch is steaming a grain in my electric pressure cooker or rice cooker. Quinoa, farro, brown rice, millet, oat groats—like my vegetables, the list of whole grains is abundant and fabulous. Again, I will have enough for several meals—breakfast, lunch, or dinner.

Let me share a little of this "good karma" with you. Picture this. At the end of the day you pull out the precooked grain, steamed veggies, a drained can of beans, and a prepared sauce. You layer everything in a bowl, what is sometimes called a "Buddha bowl," and you have dinner in ten minutes. The colors feed you visually and the abundance of micronutrients and phytochemicals feeds you nutritionally. You treat yourself to a peaceful lunch or dinner with little effort. With practice, I believe you'll experience, as I have, both greater health and heightened creativity—quite a bestowal from everyday produce.

—**Diana Tomseth**, VLCE, businesswoman
and philanthropist. EchoFund.org

8

......

Kitchen Contentment

I t's good to have a really nice kitchen. I don't mean "nice" as in "We just had our kitchen redone." I've never had a kitchen redone, unless sticking contact paper in the cabinets counts. It's just that when the place where you prepare food is welcoming and comfortable, you feel nourished before you even grab an apple.

I hope you think your kitchen is close to perfect. Mine is not. My preference would be a square kitchen, big enough for a table, with a window over the sink. But in Manhattan, people of reasonable means sacrifice preferences in order to live on an island where marvels transpire with relative frequency. Therefore, my kitchen is rectangular and compact, and has a built-in microwave that annoys me on principle. I don't microwave. I know a lot of nutrition people think it's fine and preserves nutrients and can heat food without added fat, but I find nuked food unpleasant and kind of creepy. I'd like to use that space for another cabinet, or a mirror over the stove to reflect the burners and, according to feng shui, increase my wealth. But in this compact space with its unused microwave, I prepare beautiful food for myself, my husband, and guests—sometimes a dozen or twenty or more. And I've done what I can with what's available to increase my compatibility with my kitchen.

First comes comfort. How do you feel, physically, in your kitchen?

Mine has stone floors that are as hard as, well, rock, so I have gel-core mats in front of the sink, fridge, and primary work areas. A fold-up stepstool means that nothing is out of reach. And I replaced the fluorescent ceiling fixture that made me feel out of sorts with one that uses incandescent bulbs—the full-spectrum ones to shine a happy light. (Lest you think I'm being environmentally profligate with my lighting, I'm a vegan, living in a LEED-certified green building, and we don't have a car. Even with those bulbs, my carbon footprint can't be more than a size 2.)

Feeling good in your kitchen is important because when you feel good, you want to eat well. If you're off even a little bit—you don't like the paint color, or one burner isn't working, or you've never figured out how to store pot lids in a way that doesn't irritate you when you open that cupboard—your plan to eat a Buddha bowl could turn into a doughnut hole.

Your kitchen can also help you transition seamlessly to Good Karma eating by reminding you that this is the way you do things now. If you live alone or if everyone in your household is on board with the Good Karma switch, you can do a glorious kitchen detox. This means divesting your refrigerator, cupboards, and even the area under your sink where harsh chemicals reside, of everything you now believe to be unworthy of having a place there. If you share space with people who aren't joining you in this adventure, do as much as you can to be out with the old (out with the *dead*, really). There go the animal products, and all the highly processed, chemical-laced, and sugary non-foods.

In with life! Bright, beautiful vegetables and fruits are ripening on your countertop and ready to eat in your fridge. Bananas aren't good to eat until they develop the brown freckles that tell you their hard-to-digest starch has turned to the kind of sugar your body can use and your brain is counting on. Tomatoes should never go in an icebox: store them stem-down on the counter and let them be as decorative as Christmas balls all summer and fall.

The ethylene gas produced by some fruits can help other produce ripen more quickly. The gas-producing fruits—apples, apricots, avocados, cantaloupe, figs, honeydew, nectarines, peaches, pears, plums, and tomatoes—can also hasten the demise of crisper-mates, so keep them away from ripe bananas, leafy greens, and other veggies.

You'll have comforting beans and tawny whole grains lining your pantry in glass jars—the fancy ones from a kitchen shop or equally serviceable models from Mr. Mason. More jars, these with raw nuts—walnuts, macadamias, Brazils—and seeds—flax, chia, sunflower, hemp—line the doors of your refrigerator; and both beans and seeds are sprouting on a countertop.

The Essential Art of Sprouting

Sprouting turns any kitchen into a garden, even if you're in an apartment several stories up. My favorite sprouts are sunflower, adzuki bean, and peanut. You can purchase various sprouting contraptions, but the easiest way to sprout is in an ordinary colander. Simply soak a couple of tablespoons of beans or seeds—lentils, mung beans, spicy radish seeds—in a jar of water overnight. They'll swell up some. Pour off the water, and drain your soon-to-be-sprouts into the colander (if you're using teeny-tiny seeds like alfalfa, use a fine strainer instead).

Rinse your incipient crop twice a day, jostle the colander a bit so the seeds will be slightly damp but not wet, and let them grow, with a towel beneath the colander in case there's a drip. In a day or two, you'll have baby veggies you grew yourself. Most can be eaten when there's just the hint of a sprout, but some—lentil, mung, and little sprouts such as broccoli and radish—are fine with a longer tail. Refrigerate when they're ready and enjoy them in salads; the heartier ones (generally speaking, these are bean sprouts as opposed to sprouts from seeds) can go into stir-fries or your beans-and-greens. (With the exception of chickpeas, most large beans—kidney, etc.—won't sprout in this way; neither will soybeans. Commercially grown soy sprouts, found at Asian markets, are delicious, but they shouldn't be eaten raw.)

Something happens in a kitchen when you start growing sprouts there. All of a sudden the room isn't just a repository for foodstuffs; it's a nursery for tiny, vitamin-rich plants with so much life force energy that they're the renowned mainstay of meals at respected alternative health centers, such as Hippocrates Health Institute in south Florida.

GKT

Get your children on board. Kids love sprouting—and cooking. My favorite kids' cookbooks are *Apples, Bean Dip, and Carrot Cake: Kids! Teach Yourself to Cook* by Anne and Freya Dinshah, and *Raw Recipe Fun for Families* by Karen Ranzi. Karen is also the author of *Creating Healthy Children: Through Attachment Parenting and Raw Foods*, an excellent resource for parents on a Good Karma journey.

Some experts actually make a distinction between *raw foods*—vegetables, fruits, dry nuts—and *living foods*, very young plants that are still growing, still pulsing with the energy that ignited a dormant seed and enabled it to burst forth with nothing more than a kiss of moisture. By this definition, living foods include soaked nuts and seeds, sprouts, and microgreens, tiny vegetables between the sprout stage and what is sold in stores as baby greens—adolescent greens, more like. (You can grow microgreens in a sunny window, but you will need some dirt. Check out *Microgreen Garden*, by Mark Matthew Braunstein, or Braunstein's walk-you-through-it website, MicrogreenGarden.com.)

Although I can't vouch for the accuracy of this story, I read once that some dried peas of a type believed extinct were exhumed from King Tut's tomb *and they sprouted*. Think of having this kind of liveliness in your kitchen and in your body. Sure, most of us will also have *some* packaged, convenience items, too. Buy the best brands you know of and remind yourself that, even though these products take up most of the supermarket, they play only supporting roles in a Good Karma Diet.

Jenné's Good Karma Story

. . . .

I became vegan four years ago when I realized that some of my food choices were not serving me morally. Though I was a vegetarian, and mostly vegan, before I made the commitment, I started to feel guilty each time I consumed an animal product. Eventually I had enough of it. I said so long to New York's cheesiest pizza and my daily yogurt, and then my whole world shifted.

This started unfolding just a week after becoming vegan. I'd suffered from poor digestion and stomach issues since before I can remember. As a child I was often at the doctor and missing school because of my tummy pains, indigestion, constipation, cramps, and discomfort. I had accepted this as my reality. I was born with a faulty gut. To my surprise, however, my stomach issues started going away once I stopped eating yogurt (my daily source of dairy). First the indigestion subsided, then the constipation. By the end of the second week my problems had disappeared. As my digestion improved, so did my mood, energy, and outlook. Even my ambition grew, and I became hungry for a compassionate career.

Within a year of becoming vegan, I started a personal chef service, The Nourishing Vegan, to share my passion for cooking, veganism, and nutrition, and it has become a thriving New York City company. I don't have to advertise my services, thanks to referrals and people's growing desire to eat vegan food. Cooking delicious and healthy vegan meals wasn't enough for me, though: I decided to enroll in the Institute for Integrative Nutrition to deepen my understanding of healthy eating and living. Within a year of starting the program I grew my business to include private nutrition coaching and an online program, which has become my 21-Day Vegan Blueprint eCourse.

Other doors have opened for me as well. I was invited to teach a cooking class at the Toronto Vegetarian Food Festival, the largest vegfest in North America. A month later I stood on a stage at the Cleveland Clinic speaking to over three hundred women about vegan eating. My recipes have been featured in numerous publications, and I'm now considered a vegan cooking expert.

Karma has a way of guiding us to others with a kind heart. Becoming vegan has led me to a community of other people who care deeply about the welfare of all animals, the state of health care and nutrition in this country, and the well-being of the planet. My own nana has embraced plant-based eating, lost weight, and continues to reduce her high blood pressure medications. She attributes her success to my becoming vegan. We even have big plans to collaborate on a cookbook and share our vegan cooking with the world.

If I hadn't become vegan, I would not have found the path I believe I was born to take. The food I choose to eat has shown me the importance of living with purpose. One doesn't give up happiness when they let go of cheese, steak, and sushi. It's when we accept that we are contributing to the suffering of another, and make the decision to cease doing so, that true happiness, fulfillment, purpose, and passion can enter into our lives. Good karma is waiting to bless us all.

—**Jenné Claiborne**, HHC, AADP, personal chef, blogger, and Holistic Health Counselor. TheNourishingVegan.com

9
......

Skinny Is Skinny.
Healthy Is Happy

Obesity is a scourge and a killer. It can lead to self-hatred and depression and make people miserable. It plays a role in disease and suffering and skyrocketing health care costs for which we all pick up the tab. Perhaps it's in response to this that we've made being thin a kind of holy grail, and yet our love of litheness isn't new. It appears to have started, in recent history, anyway, with the prosperity of the 1920s. Once average people had the means to fatten up, thinness, once despised as a sign of pauperdom and sickness, became desirable.

That way of thinking went underground somewhat during the Great Depression—the phrase "lean times" was literal—and during World War II, before resurfacing in the 1950s. Food was once again plentiful and there was money to buy it. Convenience and snack products had also begun to proliferate, and another part of the marketplace responded with diet pills, diet products, and "reducing salons." It was in the 1960s, however, when women sought skinny as never before, and Wallis Simpson's "A woman can never be too rich or too thin," went from sounding like "Let them eat cake" to a revered admonishment.

But there's nothing inherently healthy about being thin. You can get really thin from cancer, AIDS, anorexia, or advanced alcoholism. And thin isn't always pretty. Through your forties, extra weight tends to make you look older. After that, a little extra can make you look younger—ask any mature size zero who pays for injections from a dermatologist to plump up sunken cheeks and the backs of bony hands.

As I touched on earlier, I fought fat for thirty years. It colored my childhood and youth the drab gray of "never good enough." I've been neither overweight nor on a diet for another thirty years now, and I've worked with a lot of people who also struggle with food and body issues. We all know that the culturally correct way to address weight and dieting is to say, "It's really about health." But is it? Is this what we want? For someone who's been seriously ill, yes; that person values health above all else. But we can't just plaster a health motto onto a thin obsession and make it all okay.

No doubt about it, health is the cat's meow. In this life, it's almost everything. With it, you can make money, make babies, and make changes. You can have adventures, perform feats of valor, and strive for every hope and dream you've got. But "health" isn't sexy. It sounds like the slacker course that comes after pottery and music appreciation. Vitality and radiance, however, the earmarks of health, *are* sexy—and attractive and appealing and motivational. It's exciting that we're finally starting to accept and internalize as a culture that *strong* is indeed the new skinny.

If this is what you're after, and you have a history of what blogger JL Fields, VLCE, calls "chasing skinny" (StopChasingSkinny.com), here's what I know for sure:

- *Processed foods pack on pounds for a variety of reasons.* They lack fiber so their calories are more likely to be stored as fat. The sugar/fat combo (ice cream, cookies, pastries) and the salt/fat combo (chips, bacon, cheese) are both habit-forming:

you really *can't* eat just one. And when you eat a fractionated food that's had its nutrients stripped away through refining and high-heat processing, you're likely to feel the incessant hunger of a body starving for nutrition, even when carrying extra pounds.

GKT

Raw foods contain their full taste spectrum. Cooking dilutes flavor, encouraging us to add salt during the process. As a general rule, don't. Stick with spices and herbs as you cook, and have some lovely unrefined salt—Himalayan pink salt is my favorite—on the table.

- *To be healthy, you do need to avoid obesity, but not necessarily be "thin."* If five pounds are driving you crazy, trust me: it's not the five pounds. If you're eating a diet that's at least 90 percent unprocessed plant foods and you still have to work hard to stay at a certain weight, it may be that it's not your right weight. And if that sentence made you uncomfortable, you may be attached to thinness in a way that's impeding your ability to live fully.

- *Your body knows the size and shape it was designed to realize.* Barring some rare medical condition, if you *honestly* (I emphasize that because otherwise truthful people can lie like crazy about what they eat) adopt a Good Karma food-style and get some exercise, your body will be precisely as it's meant to be. If you don't believe that, take a hiatus from reading fashion magazines and watching awards shows.

- *Everybody has some idea about what will make you thin, and much of the time it involves something they're selling.* You don't need to engage in these discussions, whether with a friend or an infomercial. Eat plants, largely unprocessed. Don't overdo on sweets, fats, or booze. Move about because your body is a machine that has to move or it rusts. Beyond that, let all the ideas and theories and arguments about food and weight float around you, but not get to you.

- *If you eat for emotional reasons, take care of your emotions.* When life isn't rich enough in meaning and experiences, that richness has to come from somewhere else—premium ice cream and seconds on the buffet line, for instance. Except that they don't help. Therefore, do something wild and brave and important—like going vegan. Do it not to lose weight one more time, but to give your life another layer of depth and significance. Volunteer—for people or animals or somebody. Create something, starting with a beautiful meal that you eat at a table, sitting down, without a computer or a TV blunting the experience. Get a few sessions with a certified vegan lifestyle coach to learn techniques for letting food be food again, and not a mood-altering drug. If, on occasion, you want to indulge in some comfort food, make it vegan, enjoy it with someone you love, and keep right on living your amazing life.

- *If you have a serious food problem—chronic overeating, undereating, bulimia—address that before you do one more thing.* This is a bona fide addiction, like heroin or gambling or any other impasse that you can't quit and that is hell-bent on destroying your life. I personally think that Overeaters Anonymous (OA.org) is a gift from heaven, a total lifesaver. OA doesn't tell you what to eat, and it doesn't even cost money. Go there first. Stay long enough to turn your life around, and once you do you'll stay to help others. If another approach appeals, take that, but if it doesn't work, do this. Unattended, addictions are progressive. Food addiction, whether bingeing or starving, can kill you. Don't let it.

That's all. I realize that not everyone will agree with me. They'll say that weight issues are very complex, having to do with genetic and hormonal issues, the metabolic disruption that comes from repeatedly losing and gaining weight, and other factors that aren't yet understood and therefore cannot be addressed. I don't doubt that some people have weight issues because of bizarre physiological circumstances, and certainly it's important to get yourself checked out thoroughly by a physician you trust, and maybe more than one, to see if something is out of whack. Nevertheless, in all the years I've dealt with my own food issues and helped others with theirs, I've never seen anything all that esoteric. When the processed food goes, the body that processed food built goes with it.

GKT

While most of us can munch on almonds or filberts until the bowl is empty, English walnuts, already celebrated for their omega-3 content, have a stop factor built in. Four to eight walnut halves can elicit the "that's enough" response, even for those prone to overeating. (A bonus: 20 percent of the calories in any nuts aren't absorbed by the body.)

Here's the formula:

- Make peace with the body you have. Be kind to your body and caring of yourself. Love comes first, change second.

- Eat plant foods, mostly whole and unprocessed, and have some hours in the day when you don't eat at all (see chapter 10, "The Kitchen Is Closed").

- Get up and move some every day and throughout the day. If you won't do cardio, strength training, *and* stretching, do one of these until you get more in touch with your body and want to add the others.

For some people, this is a simple 1, 2, 3; for others, it's a monumental task, a commitment renewable daily, not just until they reach normal weight, but for life. If you're someone who has struggled long and hard with weight, you may feel that you just can't do it, but I'm here to tell you that you can. I certainly haven't been some perfect food goddess for thirty-one years, but I've done well enough that the weight has stayed off. If I can do it—and I was a low-bottom binger—you can absolutely do it. It may take therapy or a 12-Step Program or both. It's worth whatever it takes. As Rudolph Nureyev once said of ballet: "It never becomes easy, but it does become possible." And *possible* is pretty fabulous if you were living in *impossible* before.

The goal is not to be a body double for Audrey Hepburn or Fred Astaire. It's to feel fabulous, eat well, live long—God willing—and spend all the energy that used to go toward diet-think and self-recrimination on saving lives and ending suffering.

Philip's Good Karma Story

· ·

When I think back to who I was eight years ago, I can hardly recognize myself. My life is so completely different now that it's hard to imagine that I'm sharing the same lifetime with that man. While I have the same qualities at the core, little else about me is recognizable.

I had been overweight my entire life, tried over thirty diets, and was always the biggest kid in school. At four hundred pounds, I felt I was the victim of an obese father, a broken family, and the list goes on. The thought of giving motivational lectures and authoring books on raw food and weight loss was far removed from my reality. The only highlight of my life was my yearly vacation (escape) from work, and even that ended up being stressful. But I was soon to find out that there was much more in store for me.

Eight years ago, I switched to a 100 percent raw vegan lifestyle after going through the extensive testing process to qualify for gastric bypass surgery and then deciding against the invasive procedure. While the dramatic weight loss of over two hundred pounds resulting from my new diet was incredible for my health and confidence, what was most powerful was my new desire to live, to really live, in a way I never had before.

My new lease on life gave me the energy and clarity to take ideas that I had only imagined before and build a new vision of who I was and how I wanted my life to be. Then I got to work creating it. I always dreamed of the freedom of traveling around the world and exploring: new friends, new business partners, family, love, life. My goal was to live with as much freedom and love as my heart could handle. And today I do that.

Far too many people aren't making the most of their lives because subconsciously they don't feel they deserve anything good in life, usually due to a lack of self-love. This was how I felt eight years ago, drowning in self-disgust and depression. Now I know that I have the opportunity in every moment to create what I desire and to choose how I respond to each experience in life. I went from feeling like a victim to feeling empowered and taking responsibility for every experience in my life.

This has been the most dramatic change for me—greater even than losing over half my body weight. The weight loss and improved health was the catalyst for change, and today I am dedicated to helping others achieve vibrant health so they feel able and willing to transform their lives, too. When you have strong health and energy, you feel as if nothing can stop you. This is what continues to inspire me to do the work I do today.

—**Philip McCluskey**, speaker, author of
Raw Food, Fast Food. vimergy.com

10

......

The Kitchen Is Closed

We're nourished not by what we swallow but by what we assimilate. This means that the body has to break down the food we eat, extract the usable nutrients, and dispose of the rest. It can't do that efficiently when we're eating all day long, a relatively recent and culturally curious habit newly indigenous to North America but spreading, along with fast-food franchises, around the globe.

And yet if you've ever been a guest at a hotel or spa where meals are served on a schedule, there is great comfort in knowing when the dining room will be bustling with activity and when it and the adjacent kitchen are, simply, closed. There's likely to be a bowl of fruit left out, a pitcher of water infused with lemon or cucumber, and the makings for coffee or tea, but otherwise no one questions that between nine and noon, and two and six, it's time for pleasures that don't involve chewing and swallowing. There are lots of these, waiting to be discovered by anyone who follows one of the sanest pieces of advice ever given me: *Eat when it's time to eat, and live when it's time to live.*

Physicians and scientists and government agencies lament the obesity rates that started to balloon right around 1980. They blame TV, cars, and computers; fast food and convenience foods; soft drinks and high-fructose corn syrup; working moms and latchkey kids.

While all of these play some role, certainly, nobody brings up the coincidence that right about 1980, the *grazing* craze began.

To this day, we're often told to eat six to eight "small meals" a day. But we don't have a *tapas* mentality, so we eat two or three real meals and several substantial snacks. That's eating all day long! When you learn instead to enjoy breakfast, lunch, and dinner, all sorts of amazing things happen. Weight evaporates. Digestive issues stop being issues. You find yourself with more time, more focus (most non-mealtime eating is done while we're doing something else), and better dental checkups. (It's one thing to brush your teeth after eating three times, quite another when it's seven or eight.)

GKT

I always tell audiences: *Make your shopping cart and your plate look like a Christmas tree: mostly green with splashes of other bright colors.* Example: bright green arugula tossed with black beans, purple cabbage, red tomato, orange carrot, white radish. Different phytochemicals, the naturally occurring substances in plants that are health-promoting to us, are found in different colors of plant foods.

All you have to do to make a success of three meals a day is to eat enough at each one to tide you over. Greens and most other vegetables tend to be very low in calories, so you can eat a lot of them. This will appease your desire to taste and chew, and give your brain the twenty minutes it takes to register that you've eaten. Most people can eat fruits with relative freedom as well. Whole grains and beans have a lower water content than fruit and veg, so they're more concentrated and satisfying. They stay with you longer and, although you can eat them heartily, you'll enjoy them in smaller portions than the vegetables. Nuts, seeds, and avocado are rich in fat so you'll be eating even less of these, but the fat they contain gives a meal serious staying power.

Unless you've been diagnosed with a medical condition that requires more frequent eating, or if you're an athlete in training, or for some other reason have exceptional caloric needs, you'll be okay without solid food between meals. The body loves routine. If you're used to having lunch at twelve o'clock, you'll feel hungry at twelve o'clock. If you're used to 12:30, you'll feel hungry then. Life can interfere with your schedule—that's a sign of a full life—but have a schedule anyway.

Eating three times a day can be a boon both to health and to making peace with food if your prior relationship with it was rocky. Still, none of this came down on stone tablets. If dinner is going to be delayed, or if you're someone who experiences a really unpleasant mid-afternoon slump, tend your needs with something light and easily digestible, such as green juice, or fresh fruit and a few nuts.

GKT

When you're out with others, remember that you're being nourished by the company as well as the food, so don't worry too much if the restaurant doesn't have exactly what you were hoping for. Asian, Italian, Mexican, Ethiopian, and Indian restaurants virtually always have vegan choices; most American places have added at least one plant-based entrée; and there are always salads and side vegetables.

Ayurveda suggests that we do best by having a modest but satisfying breakfast around seven or eight in the morning; the main meal at midday (when *agni*, the "digestive fire," is hottest); and a smaller supper that ends three hours before bedtime. This way, the job of digestion is over with, so the nightly assimilation and detoxification processes can proceed unhindered. Working at a job where your lunch hour often isn't an hour, if you get to take it at all, can make adhering to this sort of structure difficult, but if you have any leeway to prioritize yourself and your health, take advantage of that. Even if your noontime meal won't be the primary one, make sure you at least have it, ideally away from your desk with a little walk after.

And when dinner is over, *get up*. Far too many people eat in front of the TV and don't budge until bedtime. The only thing worse than this would be getting up to go to the kitchen for more chips. Train yourself, gently but firmly, to eat at the table, do the dishes, and then enjoy a leisurely stroll, about ten minutes, to help your digestion.

Unless you're going out after dinner, make a plan for the remainder of the evening. If you have young children, you're likely to be involved with them. If you're on fire with some project, you'll devote yourself to that. Otherwise, can you curl up with a novel? Watch a favorite show or an On Demand movie? Play a fierce game of Scrabble with your main squeeze? Whatever it is, get involved with this in the post-supper hours and don't consume anything besides pure water or herbal tea. Rest well—I believe you will—and enjoy awakening with a keen appetite, both for breakfast and for the day ahead.

11

......

Pummeling Perfectionism

was out for lunch. Nice place, the welcoming Belgian chain Le Pain Quotidien. Not all vegetarian but highly accommodating to those of the veg persuasion. It was a sunny but unseasonably cold day in April and when I saw that the soup was butternut squash (vegan; they always have one vegan soup), my mind was made up. I ordered a large soup with whole-grain bread and a side of hummus.

Then I went to wash my hands and every table I passed was heaped with salads, lining my route as a bridal walkway is strewn with flowers. There was kale with other greens, quinoa *on* greens, lentils—on more greens. These were perfect salads, and I could just tell that the women eating them were perfect, too: attractive and smart and successful. They knew about David Mamet and Maslow's hierarchy, and they had color-coordinated closets scented with lavender sachets. "What's wrong with you?" the self-talk began. "You're supposed to be a raw enthusiast and something of an expert on matters of greenery, but you didn't order salad. And we won't even get started on your closet."

But we were about to get started on the closet and anything else that could make me feel inferior to the sachet ladies. Not wanting to go down that road, I paused, breathed on purpose, and said to myself, "Salad is good, and soup is good, and being able to eat lunch—in a restaurant, no less—is darned near spectacular. All is well, Sweetie." (I say "All is well" a lot, since at some level it's absolutely true; I just sometimes have to do some convincing to get to that level.)

The soup came, and the bread and the spread, and it was warm and comforting and pretty much all you could expect from a lunch. Truth be told, I eat a lot of greens and not so much of the orange and yellow vegetables, so the butternut squash was probably every bit as healthful for me as salad would have been. There is no "perfect" food, but any reasonably natural food you eat as a vegan can be like Baby Bear's porridge: "just right." And that's all it needs to be.

GKT

Eat at the table, even when you're by yourself. Dining in front of the TV reflects a devolution of society, in my opinion (even though I admit to being part of the degeneration some-times). Keep your dining table free from clutter—find another place for dropping mail and bags. Have candles, flowers, bright, beautiful dishes (they don't have to cost a lot), and, of course, bright, beautiful food.

We in the prosperous countries are jaded when it comes to food. There's so much of it, so many varieties, we get the idea that every meal is supposed to be a masterpiece, especially if we're dining out. In much of the world, this is not the case. I remember traveling in Nepal, riding with a driver and guide, my daughter, my boyfriend at the time, and two young girls, Tibetan refugees we sponsored, to Lumbini, birthplace of the Buddha. It was a long drive through the mountains and after several hours, I was frantic for food. We'd pass through towns and villages and our guide would say, "No food here for Westerners."

Assuming that he meant that conditions were unsanitary, I rode on with forced stoicism but finally confronted him. "What do you mean, 'no food for Westerners'?" And he replied apologetically, "Only rice and dal, ma'am, only rice and dal." Exasperated—I can get like that when I'm hungry—I said, "Tsering, that's what we eat. Please stop at the next village." We did. Admittedly, the dal was thinner than I was used to, but still aromatic and delicious.

The contrast between culinary culture in rural Nepal and middle-class America glared at me from the metal plate. If I'd gone to lunch with friends back home, somebody would have been gluten-free ("I don't have celiac," she'd say, "I just feel better without gluten"), and somebody would be oil-free ("No oil in anything or on anything"). Somebody would be off onion and garlic because her new yoga teacher had said they were irritating; someone else would be "detoxing coffee"; and I myself might have played any of these roles.

But that day, in those mountains, if I'd had any problem with rice ("Uh, this is *white* rice. That's refined. Don't you have brown?") or dal ("Beans give me gas. Can you substitute something?"), I'd have visited the Buddha's birthplace on a fast. Curiously, it was he who taught the beauty of the Middle Way. Freedom lies at that point between gluttony and deprivation, between avarice and poverty, between elation and grief. This is the place where rice and dal hits the spot, and where Baby Bear's porridge is just right. It's not perfection, but it is perfect.

Gena's Good Karma Story

I went vegan in my mid-twenties for a particular reason and with a particular goal in mind. I was suffering from terrible GI [gastrointestinal] illness, and a doctor had recommended to me that I avoid dairy in order to see if that would alleviate my symptoms. It did, dramatically, and since I was already vegetarian, I decided to remain vegan in order to keep my digestive health in order. I didn't plan on becoming an animal activist, or a food blogger, or a health care professional. I didn't plan, in other words, for veganism to shake my life up. But that's what it did, and I'm forever grateful for it.

The most profound change that's happened since I became vegan is that I've managed to enter and sustain full recovery from over thirteen years of an eating disorder. Once again, I wasn't expecting this; though nominally recovered at the time I became vegan, I was still delicate from a bad relapse, and though I professed to be moving on, I was still trapped in cycles of restriction, guilt, fear, and self-loathing. Like many people with eating disorders, I found that my inner life had become distressingly narrow, a small universe governed by tedious thoughts about what I'd eaten that day, how caloric it had been, and whether or not I had to restrain what I ate till sundown accordingly.

Veganism opened up the borders of my world again. It showed me that my food choices do not exist in a vacuum. They are part of a complex web, in which strands of environmental concern, compassion for animals, respect for my own body, and a prioritization of health and wellness come together. By choosing to eat a vegan diet, I've been able to place my food choices within a broader philosophical context, and realize that they have long-standing reverberations for other living beings.

This consciousness has transformed my previously tormented relationship with food. For better or for worse, I'm someone for whom food will always be a very big deal. But at this point in my life, it is a big deal because I recognize that it is an avenue to heal, help, and do good, and not because I use it as a means of punishing or controlling my body. Of all the good karma that veganism has brought me, this particular gift is the most meaningful. Veganism restored my body, my spirit, and my sense of purpose, and I hope that I can use them to help others who are struggling through the same terrain I once traveled.

—**Gena Hamshaw**, nutritionist, blogger, and author of
Choosing Raw. ChoosingRaw.com

12

......

Before You Feed Yourself, Nourish Yourself

You know how relationship experts say that expecting your significant other to be your everything—soul mate, psychic, shrink, shopping buddy—is asking for trouble? And yet a lot of us expect that much from food. We may ask from it not just nourishment and pleasure but consolation, stimulation, entertainment, an excuse to procrastinate, a place to chomp on our anger, and a friend who requires nothing in return. To set this—and ourselves—right, we need to be well fed before sitting down to eat.

I'm not talking about gorging on pancakes before going to the party the way Scarlett O'Hara did in *Gone With the Wind*, so she wouldn't be hungry and fail to "eat like a lady" in public. It's a different kind of nourishment—emotional, mental, spiritual—that keeps you filled up on the inside. When those parts of you are sated, you'll make the best food choices for you at any given time. Only when this is in place can you safely "listen to your body" and its food cues. Otherwise, you'll get cockeyed signals.

Oftentimes people give up on plant-based eating because they have a craving for eggs or dairy cheese, and they believe this indicates some nutritional deficit. That's not it. Cravings are most often vestiges of past loves. Tell me you've never seen a picture of an old flame and gotten fluttery all over again, even if said ex left you in misery. It's the same with food. If Grandma placated you with chocolate pudding, or your nostalgic college days were punctuated with pizza, you're going to crave those foods when you're short on comfort or excitement or some other "life nutrient" they just don't stock at Trader Joe's.

Therefore, feast on fun and binge on beauty. Relish time with family and friends. Savor sweet moments, whether with a good book, a moving film, or your dog who loves you more than anybody, except possibly your mom. The idea is to become a connoisseur of the quotidian, a doyen of the day-to-day. This means you'll be someone who walks in the rain on purpose instead of complaining about getting caught in it. You'll find more and more things interesting: nature, art, science, philosophy, your own life and everybody else's. You'll remember how to spell "boredom" but lose your ability to experience it.

GKT

Sunlight is essential. Not only does it react with your skin to create vitamin D, it's a mood-booster. Protect your face and hands with a safe sunscreen (zinc oxide or titanium dioxide), a hat, maybe even gloves, but do get outside. Indoors, I still sun-protect (glass can't block aging UVA rays), but I open the shades, have off-white walls that reflect light, and own a special lamp to simulate sunlight in winter.

Ultimately, you'll wake up almost every day feeling that your cup is running over. Before this comes about as a delightful matter of course, you can aid the process by bringing to mind ten things for which you're grateful in that virgin minute before your feet touch the floor in the morning. The more specific your list, the better. Saying "I'm grateful for Stan because he's always so positive" is better than just "I'm grateful for friends," because it's easier to envision Stan than everyone you know (not to mention the people on Facebook whom you may only sort of know). But don't fret about this: you can't do it wrong.

Gratitude is gratifying and so is human contact. Collect people—especially those who are also on a Good Karma Diet journey. It's wonderful to have people in your circle who reflect your values back to you. You know the business book *Never Eat Alone*? That's also great advice for feeling full on the inside. Every person is a world unto himself or herself, and any conversation may hold the phrase you need right now to steer your course precisely as it should go.

Nourish yourself and fill yourself with something beautiful to look at or touch or smell. Light candles for your bath and put a drop of lavender oil on your pillow. Paint a single wall red or yellow or purple. Have houseplants—ferns and ivy and mother-in-law's tongue. They'll clean the air you breathe, and one May morning an unassuming little plant just might bloom for you. On a similar note, never talk yourself out of a bouquet ("That's $7.95 and they'll just die anyway"), but think instead of Muhammad's musing: "If I had but two loaves of bread, I'd sell one and buy hyacinths, for they would feed my soul."

GKT

Engage in mindful eating. Sit down. Slow down—saying a simple table grace will bring down your speed. See your food: it's going to be pretty. Smell it. Chew it. Put the fork down between bites.

When it comes to a little blissful indulgence, my philosophy is that feeding your soul is worth any price, as long you don't go into debt to do it. Debt is metaphysically awkward: it's living in the negative column where life is unable to proceed on schedule. Therefore, be responsible with your resources, but don't cheat yourself. I've observed that too much self-denial can train life itself to get into the denial business. It's as if we say "I don't deserve" so often that the universe gets wind of it and responds with, "Well, okay, if you say so."

Surround yourself with the provisions of a full soul's larder. I need books around me, the kind with covers and paper pages. I need windows and light, and a few reminders of the life I've lived already—family pictures, travel mementos, the Buddha statue that was a gift to my first husband, who later passed away, to mark a birthday when we were both younger than our daughter is now. The statue was crafted in the thirteenth century, rescued from a demolished temple in what was then still called Ceylon, and I paid $75 for it when $75 covered half the rent. I've moved a lot. That Buddha has always been in one of the cardboard boxes.

When you're filled in the ways that satisfy your soul, satisfying physical hunger will be the simplest thing. Some salad, some broccoli, some quinoa or edamame—and maybe a bit of the bread left over after you bought the hyacinths.

Patti's Good Karma Story

My family recounts a time when I was about three years old and played with a chicken one morning on a farm where we were staying for the weekend. I talked about that chicken all afternoon. That night at dinner, I was told that the chicken I was eating was the bird I had played with earlier in the day. I would not take another bite and cried at the table.

In the following weeks I came to accept what my family told me—that some animals are to eat and some are to be our friends. Now I know better, and now I trust the instincts of children who are drawn to animals. Children know not to eat their friends.

I was in my early thirties when I became a vegetarian and then a vegan. Now I am in my early sixties. Looking back over these last three decades, it does seem that my luck—or karma—has been extraordinary. Once I started eating from the plant kingdom exclusively, my world opened up. The courage to say no to meat and dairy spilled over to other parts of my life as well. That courage enabled me to take risks that were thrilling and life changing for me and for countless other living beings.

The year I became a vegetarian, I had so much energy that I trained for and ran in the New York City Marathon, even though I'd never run more than six miles at a time before that. My fingernails got stronger, too, and I lost almost twenty pounds. Soon thereafter, I accepted a new job in California, even though I had spent my entire life until then in New York.

After two years on the West Coast, I met the love of my life, and now we've been married twenty-five years. Although I did not love the job that brought me out West, when my contract was up the courage that I'd been cultivating called me to start my own business as a literary agent. Victoria Moran was one of my first vegan clients, and she urged me to seek out others. What a sage piece of advice that was! My work and my personal life choice, to live with kindness as my guide, merged into an integrated life that I love, love, love living.

In my retirement now, I work for animal rights, human rights, and a more conscious and just world. I honor my

Jewish heritage and also study Buddhism. I helped to found Dharma Voices for Animals (DharmaVoicesforAnimals.org), dedicated to sharing Buddhist views of reverence for life and kindness to animals. In addition to courage and kindness, I credit gratitude for keeping me grounded in joy. Taking time every day to express my gratitude for so many blessings reminds me that my love and my life are large enough to include every living creature in my circle of loved ones.

My friends today sometimes have two legs, sometimes four, sometimes six, sometimes wings, sometimes scales. It feels good to have so many friends of so many kinds.

—**Patti Breitman**, speaker, animal advocate and vegan activist,
and coauthor of *Never Too Late to Go Vegan*.
www.nevertoolatetogovegan.com

13
......

Put on a Happy Plate

You know by now that I believe that eating fresh, energizing food can play an important role in keeping your spirits lifted. But into each life some rain must fall—and sometimes the basement floods. What then?

I'm convinced that what I want for dinner is a reliable indicator of my state of mind. When I genuinely want—not just think I ought to want—nutrient-dense food with lots of raw choices, you can bet that I'm pretty pleased with myself and the way my life is going. When, however, I'm drawn to less life-filled fare—packaged convenience foods, pasta but skip the *primavera*, or a vegan doppelgänger of something that made me feel better back before I knew better— there's a problem, and it's not the groceries.

This isn't a matter of wanting a treat—if you want a treat, have one—nor is it about eating out and settling, when you have to, for white-flour pasta or a dish that's richer or sweeter than you'd prefer. That's just life in a world where we don't control everything. We're looking here at what to do when you find yourself wanting food that is, let's just say, "beneath you."

This happens most often when a day isn't going well. Maybe something awful happened, but more likely your hormones are singing off-key or your stars just aren't lining up. Whatever the reason, there are likely to be mornings and evenings when you haven't the slightest interest in preparing a spread so healthy and beautiful you could turn the process into a YouTube video. No problem. You get some slack here. You have your baseline: vegan. Even if you feel wretched, you're not going to kill anybody (i.e., eat an animal). That in itself should boost your self-esteem.

There's great comfort in having a vegan foundation, an unshakeable dedication to nonviolence and peace on earth (and even having an earth, for that matter—see chapter 17, "If Mama Ain't Happy"). That foundation is with you when everything is coming up roses, and on those Eeyore-with-his-cloud days when very little seems to matter much except that this, this commitment to kindness, matters a lot, storm clouds notwithstanding.

It's a curious thing about us humans that once we set our minds to it, we can come through for others in ways we're often not able to come through for ourselves. When a woman is pregnant, for instance, she almost always eats the healthiest way she knows how for the sake of the baby. Women addicted to tobacco, alcohol, or drugs can sometimes—not always, unfortunately, but often enough to be noteworthy—lay off the harmful substance for nine full months, when they weren't able to string together nine days before. This innate altruism is so strong within us that it can provide power where none existed before.

A Good Karma Diet has this inherent altruism built in, and you can use the power it generates to help make better choices for yourself. One way to insert some dietary brightness into an otherwise dark day is to eat *something* juicy and colorful. You probably won't want it. Freshness and funk aren't naturally compatible. If, however, you can motivate yourself to eat a salad or have a green smoothie or drink some fresh juice—when you can't face making it at home, splurge at the juice bar—you'll feel better about yourself and your day. That's a promise.

GKT

Feel full two ways: first, with the stomach-filling bulk of low-fat plant foods (vegetables, fruits, legumes, whole grains); and second, with a little healthy fat (nuts, seeds, avocado, olives, and optionally some cold-pressed olive, flax, or organic canola oil) to give a meal staying power.

When I'm in the doldrums and nothing sounds good to me except macaroni and (vegan) cheese, I make mac and cheese, *but I make a salad, too, even though I have at that moment no interest whatsoever in eating salad.* I do this not for my physical health—one meal without leaves in it is unlikely to hasten my demise—but for my mental health. Having a nice salad alongside a life-looks-so-yucky-I-need-a-fourth-grader's entrée tells my brain and my cells and the universe that I care enough to eat some first-class food. I'm worth that much. The sun will come out tomorrow. And salad goes really well with mac and cheese.

Furthermore, this eat better/feel better tactic goes both ways: it can be feel better/eat better, too. Just as consuming something that says to you "Great food, great for you!" can boost your mood and self-concept, a little mood boosting can shift your food preferences. Here's what I mean: you're feeling wonky. You want a 24-ounce caffé mocha and more than one cookie. You say to yourself, "Okay, I intend to have that, but first I'm going to . . ." and then fill in the blank. Meditate, maybe. Or go for a run. Take a bath with something that smells good in the water. Send a small donation to a charity or somebody's Kickstarter campaign.

Afterward, there is a reasonable likelihood that you'll have experienced an alteration at the desire level. Maybe you'll still want the coffee but with a banana instead of the cookies. I can't cite the specifics of your transformation. I only know how transformation works, and it works by acting yourself into feeling differently. When your state of mind is different, your desires are different, too. When you feel better, your desires upgrade.

Kayle's Good Karma Story

From the age of three, I was raised on a farm in the foothills of the Sierra Nevada Mountains in Northern California. Aside from attending school, my days consisted of taking care of our animals—horses, dogs, cats, pigs, goats, bunnies, chickens, ducks, geese, cats, a sheep, and a cow. At an early age I learned to love animals, so it's no surprise that I became vegetarian the evening my cow, Cupcake, whom I'd named and hand-fed, ended up on my plate for dinner.

In high school, I became more invested in vegetarianism— I became a member of PETA and read John Robbins's *Diet for a New America*, where I learned the shocking realities of factory farming. I shopped at health food stores long before they were popular and I was often mocked for my food choices, not knowing then that something even more "extreme," veganism, would be in my future.

Just five weeks before my thirty-first birthday, and after being vegetarian for more than half my life, things changed forever. My doctor called to say: "You have cancer." The tumor in my breast was the size of a large grape. I thought I was going to die. It wasn't until I watched an array of "alternative" cancer films that I woke up to the idea of eating a 100 percent plant-based diet. Since I was in a serious health crisis, I cut out sugar, alcohol, and all junk food and became vegan at the same time. I believed plants would save me.

Following a lumpectomy to remove the tumor, I moved forward on my path to wellness without traditional Western medicine, using diet and an array of holistic treatments instead. I followed in the footsteps of my now hero, Kris Carr, the filmmaker and subject of the life-changing documentary, *Crazy Sexy Cancer*. I enrolled in a raw/living foods school, The Living Foods Institute in Atlanta, and learned everything there was to know about being a raw vegan. I chopped, I blended, I juiced, I dehydrated, I food-processed, and I wheatgrassed. I dropped thirty pounds; my skin glowed; I had lots of energy and felt amazing. Eating plants made me a happier person!

In 2009, exactly one year after my cancer diagnosis, I went in for an MRI scan, which revealed that the cancer was either back or hadn't left to begin with. I didn't let the rediagnosis get me down, though. I continued on my plant-based regime, had a unilateral mastectomy, followed by three reconstructive surgeries, four rounds of chemotherapy, and six weeks of radiation. Other than losing my hair, my body wasn't phased by any of the allopathic treatments. I was never sick. I hiked. I planted my organic garden. I thrived. In my heart of hearts, I believe I owe my success to plants.

Today, nearly six years out from my initial cancer diagnosis, I am fully recovered and totally cancer-free. I've remained vegan for my health and for the animals. I am a more compassionate person; I care more about those around me—both humans and others. My time is now spent writing a cowgirl-themed vegan blog, sharing my cancer story, and helping spread the message of health, wellness, and compassion wherever I go.

—**Kayle Martin**, blogger, speaker, and founder and Chief Cowgirl of *Cowgirls & Collard Greens*. CowgirlsandCollardGreens.com

14
......

Numbers and Letters
and Science, Oh My!

S ometimes you'll still read the old-fashioned sentence that we used to see routinely: "Vegans can have an adequate diet, but they have to be very careful to get good nutrition." Let me go on record saying that somebody standing in line at a fried chicken franchise, or waiting in the drive-thru at some burger empire, needs to be quite a bit more careful about good nutrition than the average vegan.

But first let's get clear on what we're talking about. We do ourselves no favor in seeing nourishment in a parts-and-particles fashion that ignores the complex orchestration of chemical reactions within an individual's body, and within the foods themselves, which contribute to superior health or lack of it. True, scientists have isolated substances in foods— minerals, vitamins, phytochemicals—that play various roles in health maintenance and disease prevention, but we'd be naive to assume that we know about them all. This is why real food is more valuable than the sum of its chemicals, a concept detailed eloquently in *Whole: Rethinking the Science of Nutrition*, by T. Colin Campbell, PhD, with Howard Jacobson, PhD.

An antioxidant APB: artichokes and apples, pecans and potatoes, berries and beans. Eat these foods often to prevent and repair the oxidative stress believed to lead to Alzheimer's, cancer, and heart disease.

It's curious that some people are attracted to this way of eating for ethical or aesthetic reasons but worry about what they might be "missing." Others grab on to it to, literally, save their lives. The men and women in the heart disease trials done independently by Dr. Dean Ornish and Dr. Caldwell Esselstyn Jr. are cases in point. Given up as beyond help by their cardiologists, these patients adopted a whole-food, vegan (or very nearly vegan) diet, to do something that, prior to the late 1980s, was believed impossible: reverse coronary heart disease, even in its late stages. They couldn't afford to worry about some esoteric vitamin or amino acid that a study once said vegetarians could be short on; they were in a virtual car chase with the undertaker. The positive outcomes of these studies, outcomes that translate into hundreds of saved lives, attest to the importance of big-picture health and real-world well-being over nitpicking nutritional minutiae.

On the other hand, it is a fact that certain vitamins and other named nutritional elements do exist. Some are harder to come by than others. We're going to be talking in this chapter about specific nutrients that people new to plant-based eating tend to be concerned about. In reading what follows, however, do be aware that the macronutrients—protein (comprised of amino acids), carbohydrate, fat, fiber, and water—are found in ideal amounts in plant foods, and the overwhelming majority of vitamins, minerals, and every other element needed for life and health are, too.

Thriving on a Good Karma Diet does not call for taking a boat-load of supplements. As you'll read below, every vegan needs to supplement vitamin B_{12} and probably vitamin D. According to the Academy of Medicine, however, every person over fifty ought to be supplementing with B_{12}; and physicians advise that a great many of us, excluding perhaps a few sun-worshipping surfers, take supplementary vitamin D. Supplementation with algae-based EPA and DHA (omega-3 fatty acids) may also be a prudent choice for vegans, but remember that lots of typical American eaters have been advised to take fish oil pills for the same reason. Although diet is of primary importance, the wisdom of adding a bit of something here and there as needed is not the exclusive purview of vegans.

Vitamin B_{12}

An oddity among vitamins, this one is made by bacteria and, despite what you may have read or heard, there is no reliable plant source, although plant milks, some breakfast cereals, and many brands of nutritional yeast flakes—Red Star Vegetarian Support Formula is a reliable one—are fortified with it. Failing to either consume these foods regularly or take a B_{12} supplement can lead to irreversible nerve damage, with fatigue and brain fog along the way. Lack of B_{12} can also contribute to heart disease, cancer, and macular degeneration.

You need to take only the tiniest amount of B_{12}—most other vitamins are measured in milligrams; this one is measured in *micro*grams—but you do not want to be without it. If you're under age sixty, take 100 micrograms daily. If you can get the senior discount at the movies, take 500 to 1,000 micrograms every day.

Calcium

Dark, leafy greens are full of the stuff. Of course, you have to eat (or juice) a lot of them, which high-raw, Good Karma eating suggests anyway. This has to be every day, however, and if you eat out a lot, or travel a great deal, you could come up short unless you're also including commercial plant milks (soy, almond, coconut, rice, oat, etc.) in your diet. They're fortified to have all the calcium of cow's milk, and in some cases, 50 percent more. Other very good sources include blackstrap molasses and tofu cultured with calcium sulfate; almonds, broccoli, and tahini also have a decent amount of calcium.

Vitamin D

This is a vitamin that becomes a hormone. You need it for bone health, and deficiency has been linked to depression, weight gain, frequent colds, and several types of cancer. We're supposed to get vitamin D from sunlight, but if you live in the north or wear sunscreen (I do both), that won't be happening. Perhaps this is why, in recent years, almost everybody seems to have become deficient in vitamin D. Or maybe they weren't testing for it properly before, or the current test is ultra-sensitive and shows deficiencies where none exist. Because I don't know—and no one else seems all that sure, either—it seems wise to get your levels checked and follow the advice of a physician you trust.

Nondairy milks and margarines are fortified with vitamin D just as cow's milk and butter are, but there's not much there. The RDA (recommended dietary allowance determined by the Food and Nutrition Board of the National Academy of Science's Institute of Medicine) is 600 IU (those are International Units, a measurement used for certain vitamins based on biological activity rather than weight). However, individual needs may vary widely. Although it's theoretically possible to get too much, taking 1,000 IU daily is believed to be safe, and your doctor may recommend that you take more. Vitamin D_2 is the type that comes from plants. Vitamin D_3 almost always comes from animals—from fish oil or from lanolin, a derivative of wool. Vitamin D_2 is now believed to be as effective as vitamin D_3 as long as you take it every day. If you tend to skip some days, look for a vegan vitamin D_3 supplement, such as Vitashine.

Iodine

Iodized salt is the most reliable source of this thyroid-protective trace mineral. It was first added to salt when there was a virtual epidemic of goiter, a sign of severe iodine deficiency, in the Northern United States. Eating sea vegetables on a regular basis should also meet your needs. If in doubt, consider a supplement of 90 micrograms a few times a week.

GKT

Sea vegetables are an excellent source of iodine and other minerals. Avoid hiziki (sometimes spelled hijiki)—it picks up arsenic from polluted waters; and limit kelp to the little flakes you'd use as a salt substitute: kelp is so high in iodine you could overdose on this trace mineral. Dulse, nori, alaria, and wakame are safe, healthy seaweeds.

Iron

The iron in plant foods is less absorbable than that in meat, which is good news for men and postmenopausal women for whom excess iron may contribute to heart disease, dementia, or (for the men) prostate cancer. Women of childbearing age who are prone to iron deficiency can up their intake by including blackstrap molasses in their morning smoothie, and also by eating legumes of all sorts, leafy vegetables including bok choy and kale, whole grains such as bulgur wheat and millet, watermelon, and dried fruits (raisins, prunes, apricots)—there's lots of iron in their soaking water, too. Using cast-iron cookware can contribute to iron stores, as will consuming a food rich in vitamin C—lemon juice is easy—with iron-rich foods to enhance absorption.

Omega-3 Fatty Acids

Being in good fatty acid status—having enough of the hard-to-get omega-3s and not too much of the ubiquitous omega-6s—appears to decrease inflammation in the body; protect against depression, notably postpartum depression; and help guard against heart disease and dementia. Avoiding processed foods and most polyunsaturated oils—safflower, sunflower, almond, corn, etc.—is a good way to keep your omega-6 intake in check. Plant sources of omega-3 include flaxseeds, chia seeds, soy foods, and walnuts.

However, the omega-3 from plants, ALA, must be converted to EPA (this is done pretty well) and DHA (this doesn't proceed as smoothly) for use in the body. The solution appears to be to eat some omega-3-rich plant foods every day, knowing that at least a portion of it is converted to a usable form; and consider taking an algae-based (vegan) omega-3 supplement providing 250 milligrams of DHA several times a week. The brand I take is nuIQue—they're the smallest caps I've found.

Protein

This is the one to worry about least, but you'll be asked about it most. Protein is in every whole, plant food. It's really impossible to become deficient in protein unless you aren't getting enough calories to maintain a normal weight; or you consume so much junk food and/or alcohol that you're excluding most other foods; or if you attempt to live on nothing but fruit, which has only a little protein, while vegetables, legumes, whole grains, most seeds, and some nuts have quite a bit. All the amino acids are found in a varied, plant-based diet, so you don't have to combine certain foods to cover your bases. Just be sure to eat some legumes—beans, lentils, dried peas, soy foods (tofu, tempeh, soymilk), or peanuts daily for lysine, an amino acid that can be somewhat elusive otherwise. (Pistachios and quinoa also contain substantial lysine, so Virginia Messina, MPH, RD, calls them "honorary legumes.")

Selenium

Brazil nuts are an excellent source of this trace mineral. One a day—or, more precisely, twenty-two a month—will take care of your selenium needs. (Avoid selenium supplements—it's easy to get too much.)

Zinc

Essential for immune function, zinc is richly supplied in pumpkin and chia seeds, but you'd need to eat a lot of them to get the RDA. There is also some conjecture that vegetarians need extra since zinc from plant sources may be difficult to absorb. A supplement of 15 to 30 micrograms per day (or a higher amount a few times a week) may be helpful.

Just When We Thought It Was OK$_2$ Go Back in the Kitchen . . .

Vitamin K, which helps in blood clotting and calcium assimilation, is found abundantly throughout the plant kingdom, so vegans never worried. Then we started hearing scuttlebutt about vitamin K$_2$, believed to be necessary for bone strength but found only in animal foods and a fermented soy product called *natto*—an acquired taste at best and downright disgusting to most Western palates. Some studies have suggested that everyone should consume K$_2$, which is available as a fully vegan supplement. However, a preponderance of conflicting studies show that vitamin K$_2$ can indeed be synthesized from vitamin K$_1$ and we can go back to not worrying.

Are you confused yet? Me too. I have a bottle of vitamin K$_2$ in my cupboard and take one when I think of it, a couple of times a week probably. Maybe that's better than nothing, and maybe it's overkill. In my long observation of people who are vibrantly healthy and those who are not, the ones who eat real food and show real love do the best. You can't fit either one of those in a gel cap.

While other nutritional supplements may be valuable when prescribed for some therapeutic purpose, when it comes to simply fulfilling your nutritional needs, you're pretty well educated right now. Nutrition is a relatively new and still inexact science. While experts debate the fine points, headlines report on the latest, definitive, and ultimate study, more often than not because it contradicts the last splashy study. Good nutrition shouldn't be this complicated. The squirrels in my building's courtyard and the rabbits who love whatever is coming up in your garden apparently get by all right doing what comes naturally.

Modern life is far from natural, but we are rational, or at least we can be, and we need to apply this rationality to our food choices. The environmental crisis alone demands that thoughtful men and women withdraw their support from animal agriculture. We need to do this with good sense, meaning that we eat a variety of minimally processed foods from the plant kingdom, and that we take vitamin B_{12} regularly and perhaps a few other thoughtfully selected supplements. That may not be sexy enough for a headline, but it's simple, and its effect can be profound.

If you're working with some preexisting pathology or you have some special dietary circumstance that needs to be addressed by a licensed professional, consult with a registered dietitian who's well-versed in plant-based nutrition and, ideally, understands your commitment to this choice. Find such a wonderworker through the Vegetarian Nutrition Practice Group of the American Academy of Nutrition and Dietetics (formerly the American Dietetic Association). Go to vndpg.org and click "Find a Registered Dietitian."

If you're not in the market for one-on-one counsel but you'd like to learn more about plant-based nutrition, excellent books include *Becoming Raw* and *Becoming Vegan*, both by Brenda Davis, RD, and Vesanto Melina, MS, RD; and *Vegan for Life*, by Jack Norris, RD, and Virginia Messina, MPH, RD. It shouldn't take too many books to make us as smart as the squirrels and the bunnies.

15
......

Animal Stories

What's your animal story? Nearly everybody has one, and most of us have several, usually involving a companion animal. I have one about Nell, my first dog. She hadn't always been my dog, though. She originally belonged to my maternal grandfather, and I'd often heard the tale of Nell's saving his life during the attempted burglary of his little gas station on a county highway. This lifesaving feat probably entailed her hearing the intruders and barking, but the story had been so heavily embellished that by the time I came along, I knew Nell as a canine superhero, fully prepared to risk all for those in her charge.

When my grandparents' health deteriorated and they could no longer care for Nell, she moved in with us. She was sixteen and I was six, in first grade at a private girls' school in Kansas City. My parents had both made their way out of hardscrabble childhoods into successful careers; they could easily pay the tuition, but we so did not fit in. I wasn't aware of that at six, and it seemed reasonable to me to enter Nell, despite her lack of "papers," in the annual dog show.

Our competition included poodles with hair bows, an imposing Great Dane, and a broad bulldog named Winston, as so many are. Nell and I found our place and, on cue, proceeded to walk the circuit before the judges. After a couple of minutes, she got tired and opted to sit a spell. There we were: an ancient, arthritic mutt with short black hair and soulful eyes, and a chubby little girl with an unfortunate perm, who was yet to learn that in the eyes of this august company, she had no more "breeding" than her dog.

Had it been fifth grade instead of first, I'd have been mortified by Nell's impromptu time-out, but I was still young enough to accept things at face value: she was tired and needed to sit. What's wrong with that? When she was ready to walk again, we finished the route and waited for the judging with the other K-through-second girls and their dogs, who smelled strangely like—perfume? I wasn't sure.

The results were in: first, a slew of honorable mentions. That sounded so important, being honorable. We didn't get one. Then third place—yellow ribbon. Second place—red (I remember to this day that the Great Dane got that one). "First place in the K-through-Second Division goes to Nell, and her handler, Vicki Mucie." I was overcome with pride: we won! They knew Nell was a heroine and a dog among dogs.

In retrospect, I'm sure the awarding of that blue ribbon was an uneasy act of charity, but my dog was a champion nonetheless. She stood for pride in who you are, sticking up for those you love, and sitting down when you're tired because it just makes sense. Nell shaped my character. So did Billy, the dog who came next, a white—except when my mom had the grooming lady tint him pink—standard poodle. I was influenced, too, by the cats we hid from the landlords after my parents' divorce, and the injured pigeons and sparrows we tried to save.

GKT

Most dogs can be happy and healthy on completely vegetarian diets, using either commercially available food—brands include V-Dog, Ami Pet, and Evolve—or homemade fare. For recipes, see *The Simple Little Vegan Dog Book*, by Michelle Rivera.

In adulthood, my first animal companions were two white mice, Clementine and Priscilla, and then the cats: first, Benjamin, Henry, and Albert (I named them for famous vegetarians—Franklin, Thoreau, and Schweitzer—even though they were felines and carnivores). Later, Bobby came. This was when I was a single mom and we named Bobby for Bob, my boyfriend at the time, a man who cared about animals in general but wasn't crazy about pets. I thought that having a namesake might help.

Then someone new entered our lives, the scared and skinny stray bird dog I lured into my car with cat food from a recent supermarket run. I intended to find her the proverbial "good home," but my daughter, then eleven, took one look and said, "I'm going to name her Aspen because we were in Aspen when you said I could have a dog." That was two years earlier. I'd forgotten. She hadn't.

An aging Aspen went to live with Adair when she got married, and Bobby, our last surviving cat, stayed with William and me, living to eighteen. After Aspen and Bobby died, it look a while for me to open up to another four-pawed companion, but when I saw a scruffy black schnauzer-poodle-and-maybe-something-else in a cage on adoption day at Petco, it was time. That's Forbes, here and now, world's best dog. Of course, they're all the world's best dog—and cat and horse and gerbil and turtle and parakeet and goldfish. We know *this* because we've known *them*.

Very few of us get to know a cow or pig or chicken. We don't have the opportunity to learn firsthand that any one of them could be the world's best, too. And yet these beings are fully aware of themselves and their surroundings, and they are emotionally and intellectually complex. Not only are they sentient, fully capable of feeling both pain and pleasure, but they form bonds with members of their own species and with us, and they remember past experiences.

Even so, to provide some of us with franks and shakes and buffalo wings, and others with broiled chicken, grilled salmon, egg white omelets, and nonfat yogurt, we slaughter these individuals by the billions and torture the vast majority mercilessly throughout the days, months, or years of their truncated lives. We tend to ignore what happens to them because it's too awful to contemplate. But if it's too awful to contemplate, it's too awful to support.

GKT

Language is powerful. Refer to nonhuman animals as "he" or "she" instead of "it." Replace a phrase like "more than one way to skin a cat" with "more than one way to peel a carrot."

The next chapter is a brief overview of what happens to animals raised for food. I realize it's unpleasant and a lot of people will skip over this part. Believe me, I don't want to write about the way these animals suffer any more than you want to read it. But just as hiding human atrocities and genocides doesn't make them go away, keeping this evil out of sight and out of mind only perpetuates it.

If you no longer consume animal products, or you've eliminated many and you're on your way to eliminating more, and if you're sufficiently educated about animal agriculture that you can answer the questions you'll be asked, you've earned the right to move past chapter 16. But if you support the meat, poultry, egg, dairy, or fishing industries with your purchasing power, or if you've stopped but don't know how to respond to someone who says, "They don't have to kill the cow to get the milk," or "I eat only 'humane' meat," please learn a few salient facts. These will empower you as an advocate for those who can't speak for themselves, and enable you to better make decisions about the food that will comprise your very cells, and the world you want for yourself and your children.

Sarah's Good Karma Story

I went vegan when I was fourteen, half a lifetime ago. The decision for me was an easy one. I was a sensitive kid, to a fault, but I hadn't been raised a vegetarian. Growing up, there was a pool in my backyard. I'd check the skimmer daily for frogs (or snakes!) that may have accidentally found their way in. To discover them too late would always mean a funeral scene behind the pool. Frogs were my special pals— seeing a tiny tree-hugger stuck to our kitchen window while I ate breakfast was the exciting push I needed to head out for a good day of school. So when it was revealed one evening at the dinner table that my sister's science class had been dissecting frogs all week, I put down my fork and lost it! And I realized immediately that meat wasn't necessary for me. I gave up eating animals at age ten.

A few years later, while reading a book on healthy vegetarianism for teens, I learned about the horrendous world of factory farming. I transitioned from partially to fully vegan within the next few months. Being such a young vegan adopter, I didn't notice much difference in my energy level or well-being, as I think children are automatically more energetic and spiritually connected to the natural world. But over the next few years, I saw negative changes in my peers that I didn't have to deal with.

Case in point: I was training to be a professional ballet dancer. I was happy as a clam to start rehearsing when the sun rose and continue until after it set each day. It was a little embarrassing to have so much more energy than my fellow dancers, eschewing the breaks they begged for. I definitely got friendly jibes for messing with the "curve" of what was humanly possible. I attribute my stamina to my clean way of eating. I relied on nut butters for sustained energy with no crash. My friends were still into the fast-food and SAD (Standard American Diet) thing, which they thought was cool—they were able to eat what celebs in commercials promoted—but it certainly wasn't helping them for the long haul.

Today my diet serves me in a different way. I realized that a career in ballet wasn't going to help the animals in my midst, suffering silently. So when I moved to New York City eight years ago, I let my emotions rule. It was not ballet auditions that sucked me in. Instead, I was drawn to the world of vegan chocolates, just beginning to take off with single-origin beans and innovative processing concepts. I was inspired every time chocolate hit my tongue.

Not long after my happily exhaustive survey of the NYC chocolate scene, I began my own company. My chief inspiration was animal rescue in general and, more specifically, the rescue of my first dog, a special pit bull named Mocha. Today, Rescue Chocolate spreads the animal rescue message through the sweetest and most delicious vessel I know. It has been humbling to see the stupendous response from customers, and inspiring to help skeptics realize that no milk is needed to make a sublime chocolate.

—**Sarah Gross**, president, Rescue Chocolate, and coproducer of
the NYC Vegetarian Food Festival. RescueChocolate.com

16

......

Do Unto Others

This guy walks into a bar. Seriously—the guy was my husband, William, who sat a few stools down from a friendly salesman in his forties, who was eating a sizable Reuben sandwich and drinking a vodka tonic. William ordered a salad and a glass of Merlot, and the other fellow started a conversation:

"Why are you eating salad?"

"Because I'm vegan."

"Oh, I should do that, too. I know eating meat is bad for me."

"It's even worse for the meat."

The guy with the Reuben looked perplexed, maybe because, as William later learned, this was his *fourth* vodka tonic. But it's so simple. You or I could eat some meat in moderation and we'd probably be all right, but there's no moderation for "the meat," the individual whose life, almost assuredly miserable, was sacrificed for a sandwich.

It happens 285 times a second. That's how often, in the United States alone, someone is slaughtered because he or she is considered to be a "food animal." And this doesn't even include the fishes whom we kill in vastly greater numbers.

Please don't take my word for any of this. Do your research. I'd suggest that you visit a slaughterhouse, a factory farm, and a fish farm for yourself, but that's as difficult as attempting to take a stroll through Fort Knox. These places have become increasingly off-limits in recent years. In some half-dozen states (as of this writing) it's illegal for an undercover whistle-blower to apply for a job at one of them, and in some cases, you'd break a law to either enter or photograph a farmed animal facility.

There are some laws on the books protecting farmed animals, but those in the United States, at least, contain mammoth loopholes and often exclude "customary agricultural practices." The more draconian practices become customary, the more horrors become legal.

The following is a surface citing of a few undeniable and easily vetted facts about the state of animals raised for food. There's a great deal more to learn. If you want that information, there's some in my earlier book, *Main Street Vegan*; and more in Jonathan Safran Foer's richly written account *Eating Animals*; and in *Farm Sanctuary: Changing Hearts and Minds About Animals and Food*, by Gene Baur, cofounder of Farm Sanctuary. Gene holds a master's degree in agricultural science from Cornell University, and he has personally witnessed more farmed animal abuse, and more abused animal rescues, than probably anyone I know. For now, here are five areas to consider, just what you can count on the fingers of one hand.

GKT

Purge your library. Go through your diet and nutrition books and get rid of the ones that are crazy about animal products or down on vegetarians. Your transition will be easier if you tune out dissenting voices for now by getting these titles off your bookshelf or out of your e-reader. Once you're grounded in your new choice, you can read what others are claiming without being discombobulated by it.

Separation

We tend to eat animals whose species are, like our own, gregarious. They gather in flocks, herds, or schools, and many form strong family ties, notably the mother/child bond. These social systems and family units are severely impeded in the "factory farming" model that provides some 98 percent of animal foods. A mother pig is restrained (see section 3 of this chapter, "Confinement") during the nursing period and cannot bond with her piglets, who are removed after early weaning so she can be impregnated yet again.

Dairy cows suffer obvious agony—crying, often for days—when their babies are removed, commonly within twenty-four to seventy-two hours of their birth. The orphaned calves are fed formula so we can take the milk. Baby girls may be kept for the same cycle of impregnation, birth, kidnapping, and grief as their mothers, but if they're not needed for dairying, they go to auction where, like the boys, they'll likely face either immediate slaughter (infanticide seems to be the word that fits) or live a few months as veal calves before their death.

Mutilation

In a factory farm environment, it's evidently believed that God doesn't know how to make an animal, because pigs—who are, incidentally, smarter than dogs and three-year-olds—have their ears docked, their tails cut off, their testicles removed, and their teeth pulled out or ground down—all without anesthesia.

Chicks in egg operations, and sometimes those being raised for meat if they're being used as "breeders," have the sensitive tissue of their beaks sliced through, often on two occasions, so they won't peck their fellow prisoners. Both "broilers," the chickens people eat, and turkeys have been bred with breasts so large that, if allowed to reach maturity, they can have trouble walking.

Cattle are branded with hot irons, and beef and dairy cattle are routinely de-horned, without anesthesia. The testicles of beef cattle are bound with a tight band that causes them to "rot off." (Every man I know who hears this gets a sick look on his face. The "real men" among them never eat another burger, unless it's veggie.)

Confinement

It's right there in the industry's own terminology: CAFO, *Confined Animal Feeding Operation*. It's the post–World War II version of the idyllic barnyard: hidden away in barracks instead of barns, where torture, some illegal, some "customary," is commonplace. The worst offender is probably the battery cage for egg production, and public opinion is overwhelmingly on the side of banning these dens of over-crowding, suffering, insanity, and death. A CAFO "chicken farm" is also a great breeder of disease, the primary reason citizens' groups are periodically up in arms about the antibiotics routinely fed to poultry.

"Barren" battery cages, which afford each bird less space than a sheet of paper and lack any "enrichments" such as wood shavings or perching space, have been outlawed by the EU, California, Michigan, Oregon, and Washington; Ohio has legislation preventing the introduction of new barren battery cages. Most of this legislation does not demand a cage-free, much less free-range, situation, however. In most cases, the replacements are "colony cages"—12 by 4 feet, an improvement for certain, but a good life for chickens? Hardly.

Gestation crates for pigs vie for the dubious distinction of "worst" atrocity. A mom-to-be is held virtually motionless throughout her repeated pregnancies in "gestation crates" that call to mind an invention of the Inquisition. After giving birth, she's again held captive in a "farrowing crate" for nursing, until the cycle begins again. "This perpetual immobilization lasts for years on end," says Paul Shapiro, vice president of Farm Animal Protection for the Humane Society of the United States.

Some veal calves in the United States and Canada are still enclosed in barbaric crates so small that they are unable to turn around, but due to public outcry and relentless pressure from animal protection organizations, more than 70 percent are now housed in groups, not crates. Beef cattle are not confined until their grazing lives end and they're sent to vast, arid feedlots to be fattened on corn, a substance so unsuited to their digestive systems that an excess can cause a bovine stomach to literally explode.

Approximately half the fish eaten in the United States and worldwide are "farm raised" and suffer the same kind of confinement on, arguably, an even more severe scale. Undercover footage has shown filthy conditions on many infiltrated fish farms, and some supermarkets touting their salmon and other fish as "wild-caught" have been found to be lying outright.

It's the horrors of confinement that send many consumers looking to "small, local farms" for something better. They are indeed better. If you're transitioning away from animal foods, purchase the ones you still eat from these providers. Do not, however, kid yourself that this is a solution.

Unless you visit a farm yourself—ideally, unannounced—you don't know what goes on there. Labels on eggs, for instance, that read "cage-free" or "free-range" can mean almost nothing, certainly not that the hens are outdoors pecking and roosting and engaging in the normal social behaviors of their species. The meat, eggs, and dairy products from exemplary local farms are prohibitively expensive for most families, and even people who routinely eat this kind of food at home still support factory farming, unless they order only vegan meals when they dine out.

Small farmers are able to raise animals without the extreme

confinement of the factory system, but they're still in business, and in the business of agriculture, animals are production units. Branding, castration, killing of sick or unwanted specimens, and the separation of dairy cows from their babies (although usually at a later date than in the factory system) take place on small farms, too.

Transport

The U.S. law covering the transport of farmed animals was drafted in 1873. As hard as it is to believe, that's not a typo. There have been revisions, of course, but the crux of this antediluvian statute, known as the 28-Hour Law, remains. "It says that farm animals cannot be transported more than twenty-eight hours without five hours of food/water/rest in between," explains Shapiro. "And, alas, USDA interprets the law to exclude poultry, ninety-five percent of all land-based farm animals."

Laws change because times change, but laws protecting animals change slowly. There is suffering in transport. Animals are virtually never provided with food or water on their journey to slaughter and, for cattle, from pasture to feedlot. Frightened animals are usually loaded into crowded, open truck cars in all weather conditions. Some die on the trip, and those who arrive at slaughter too weak or ill to walk may be left to perish on "dead piles."

Toronto Pig Save (TorontoPigSave.org) is one grassroots organization, within a larger developing SAVE movement, formed to bring public awareness to the cruelty inherent in farmed animal transport and the rest of the meat business. Members manage to show some modicum of compassion to truckloads of pigs who pass through a particular intersection in the capital. "We had to work hard at being unemotional when they went by," says Stephanie Gorchynski, VLCE, one of the early participants in this effort. "We needed to offer love and light to those trucks—the animals and the drivers." Volunteers give water and a loving touch through the trucks' bars to thirsty, terrified animals. It's a tiny gesture, given all they've endured, but given all they've endured, it's likely the first kindness they've known on earth.

Killing

Essentially every animal in agriculture, unless they die of some injury or illness first, is killed—most often by the slaughterer's knife or, in the case of fish, suffocated on a line or in a net. Some are deemed as having no value and subsequently get no taste of life at all— newborn boy chicks in egg industry hatcheries, for instance. And the unwanted fish, sea mammals, and sea birds caught in giant trawlers die because they're "by-catch," unneeded, unnecessary.

There may be someplace worse than a slaughterhouse, but I haven't been there. I spent one day in a slaughterhouse back before they became top-secret enclaves, going to extreme lengths to hide their daily business from the curious and from the consumers of their products. I was required to outfit in surgical garb as if entering some sterile environment, but the smell of blood and death clung to the clothing underneath so that after several worthless washings, I had to throw it all away.

The place felt icy—it was refrigerated, after all—and the workers were relegated to the status of automatons, mere machines set to stunning, slitting, butchering, all for low wages and the highest injury risk of any job that OSHA tracks. The plant I toured—I pretended to be a home economics grad student—"processed" only cows and pigs, animals required by law to be stunned prior to slaughter. Kosher and halal plants are exempt from this protection, and chickens, turkeys, ducks, and geese are left out entirely, even though the science is clear that birds are as sentient as any mammal, including us.

You Can Come Back Now

If you opted to skip the paragraphs above, welcome back.

These are facts, and I don't cite them to make anybody feel guilty. Very few of us were born vegan. I supported these industries before I knew better, and even after, when I held on to eggs and cheese like a junkie to his needle, my dollars helped the atrocities persist.

I also don't include this information to shock you into making an emotionally fueled one-eighty that you can't sustain. There's a telling quotation from Oscar-nominated film director Jason Reitman: "Most people see a documentary about the meat industry and then they become vegetarian for a week." If you can make a total change-over and stay totally changed, excellent, but flashing in the pan hardly makes a dent. Start where you are and do what you can do. Celebrate the lifesaving power of every incremental step, and keep moving forward.

Adopt a rescued, formerly farmed animal at a sanctuary. This doesn't mean you'll take a cow or goat into your home. Instead, you'll help pay for that animal's life at the sanctuary, allowing the organization to continue its work in both rescue and public education. An abbreviated, alphabetical list of the many doing wonderful work in the world includes:

- Catskill Animal Sanctuary (New York)

- Cedar Row Animal Sanctuary (Ontario)

- Farm Sanctuary (New York and California)

- For the Animals Sanctuary (New Jersey)

- Ironwood Pig Sanctuary (Arizona)

- Peaceful Prairie Sanctuary (Colorado)

- PIGS, a Sanctuary (West Virginia)

- Pigs Peace Sanctuary (Washington)

- Tower Hill Stables Animal Sanctuary (Essex, UK)

- Vine Sanctuary (Vermont)

- Woodstock Farm Sanctuary (New York)

Once you adopt an animal at a sanctuary, you forge a relationship with some*one* you may have thought of before as merely some*thing*. "Your" pig or chicken or cow will be the ambassador, helping you know through and through that these beings are no longer abstractions but friends, just like the companion animals who've made you laugh and given you love.

Learn what you need to learn and get the support you need to stay with your dietary revisions. Be sure your food is delicious and satisfying. Have fun poring over cookbooks and viewing food prep videos until you have a repertoire of dishes you'll look forward to preparing and serving. We're on the brink of an evolutionary leap to respect for all beings. You're at the forefront. Remind yourself of this very big picture whenever there's not much to choose from on a menu.

Russell's Good Karma Story

I have had cancer twice. When I was a boy, thirteen years old, a malignancy required that my left arm be amputated. Never mind that I was left-handed. Never mind that the chemo almost killed me as much as the tumor itself. I survived. At the time my family lived on ten acres of land in rural Texas, and some friends from church gave me two cows who had two babies. I loved those cows, fed them, cared for them, and played with them. When it came time to sell the cows, like you did in rural Texas, I was heartbroken and decided I'd become a vegetarian.

It didn't last long initially, but the idea of being kind to animals kept coming back again and again. In college and graduate school I studied religious ideas and counseling. I was a committed vegetarian by then and thought I was doing a good deed each time I sat down to eat. Never mind that I was heavier than I'd ever been, or that my cholesterol was continually moving upward, or that I simply didn't feel so good.

Then, I got cancer again, this time in the rectum—good ol' butt cancer. Once more the doctors brought out their knives and carved me up. They permanently changed the way my body works. They radiated me and filled me with pills that made me tired and sick.

You are never so out of control as when you are in the hospital. You eat when told; you sleep when told (only then to be told to wake up); you bathe when told; you take your medicine when told. I don't like being sick and I don't like being told what to do. So I started reading and reading and then read some more. I came across a way of eating that was even kinder to animals than vegetarianism is, and there was no doubt it was better for me, too. I became vegan! No flesh, no eggs, no dairy, nothing that came from an animal.

I found supporters in my religious community. I found answers to my questions on nutrition and wellness. I can certainly say, as I look back on my early days of veganism, I'd found a new way of life, a new way of living. Never mind that I lost around fifty pounds. Never mind that my blood pressure normalized and my cholesterol dropped dramatically. Never mind that I have rarely been sick since making the decision to eat in a way that was life altering and life affirming.

The karmic surprise was that I could look into the eyes of other beings and know that, as best I could, I would not contribute to their harm or the harm of their species. I was kinder. I was gentler with all souls, including my own. It is still a journey. I am not perfect by any stretch of the imagination. But I am a better person today and am still becoming. I went into the ministry to further the well-being of all people. Now, I am focused on the well-being of all beings.

—**Russell Elleven**, DMin, VLCE, clergyman. MinisterOfHealth.org

17

......

If Mama Ain't Happy

You've heard the phrase applied to family life: "If Mama ain't happy, ain't nobody happy." There's a bigger picture, though, and a much bigger Mama. Mother Earth, who provides the stage setting for all natural history and human history, has not been happy for quite some time.

The environmental mess we're in is complex and distressing. It's full of numbers and statistics and parts per million, places where the left-brained love to play and which I attempt to avoid like a dangerous neighborhood. But the real off-putter is that one of our environmental problems could drastically change life on earth as we know it, and do so in our lifetimes. We're talking, of course, about climate change, unfortunately dubbed "global warming" so naysayers can shout "Told ya so!" every time there's a cold snap.

I know that a phrase like "change life on earth as we know it" sounds alarmist to the point of absurdity, like those doomsday prophets who knew for certain when the world would end, except it didn't. In this situation, however, the overwhelming consensus among top scientists is that climate change is a present reality and imminent peril. And its number one human-induced cause—not the only one, but far and away the most impactful—is raising animals for food in the numbers we do today.

This is a complete surprise to most people, even avowed environmentalists. What have we all been told to do to be good stewards of the earth? Reduce, reuse, recycle. Replace your car with a smaller one, preferably a hybrid, and drive less. Switch to energy-efficient appliances. Use less heat and A/C. If food comes up at all, it's a reminder to stick as closely as possible to what's locally grown. This is all helpful, the way it's helpful for a smoker with a lung disease to do breathing exercises and have houseplants. But it's essential that a person with a lung disorder *stop smoking*—this very instant or, preferably, yesterday. And it's essential that a planet with a climate disorder *stop breeding so many animals for food*—preferably yesterday, but ASAP will have to do.

Animal agriculture contributes somewhere between 14 percent (UN figure) and 51 percent (World Bank Group figure) of the greenhouse gases emitted into the atmosphere because of human activity. *All transportation combined comes in at only 13 percent.* And the major climate-degrading gas produced by animal agriculture is methane, which, if output were drastically curtailed, could leave the atmosphere in about ten years. If we saw, instead, the hypothetical cessation of carbon emissions, that greenhouse gas would take somewhere in the neighborhood of one hundred years to dissipate.

"Surely, we must deal with overpopulation, overconsumption, and the burning of fossil fuels, but these tasks will take many decades, if not centuries," says *Healthy Eating, Healthy World* author J. Morris Hicks. "Dealing decisively with food choices *now* may buy us the time we need to address these other issues." Another heartening ramification of a significant decrease in animal agriculture would be that this shift would allow vast amounts of land to be reforested; the trees would decrease the amount of carbon in the atmosphere.

Go to the movies. Veg-friendly documentaries are fabulous! To learn about animal ag and the environment, check out *Cowspiracy*, and for health and ethics and all the rest: *Earthlings, Fat, Sick & Nearly Dead, Forks over Knives, Game Changers, The Ghosts in Our Machine, May I Be Frank, Speciesism: The Movie, Vegucated, PlantPure Nation, Peaceable Kingdom: The Journey Home, Simply Raw: Reversing Diabetes in 30 Days,* and *Unity.*

The call to action, then, is to go vegan, or at least cut back drastically and permanently on consuming meat and other animal products. "We have the greatest opportunity anybody has ever had to get healthy, be happy, save money, and save the planet. I don't know why we don't choose that," says Terry Gips, cofounder and president of the Alliance for Sustainability. And this simple adjustment can do so much so quickly. For example, a Carnegie Mellon University study found that eating vegan once a week prevented more greenhouse gases from entering the atmosphere than eating locally grown food for a full year.

The Atavistic Act of Raising Animals for Food

I think I learned the word "atavistic" from watching *Jeopardy!*, or maybe reading the *New York Times*. Either way, it describes something that's reverted to the ancient or the ancestral. In biology, it can refer to an evolutionary throwback, or in sociology to a society's returning to practices and mores of an earlier era. There's no better adjective for eating animal products and raising animals for food at this time in history. We've done it for a long time. When there weren't a lot of people on the planet, it worked pretty well (not for the animals, but that's another chapter). The animal manure fertilized the fields. Crops grew. And we did a whole lot of fruitful multiplying.

But the human population explosion has led to a far larger and even more unsustainable explosion in the farmed animal population. Eating meat is atavistic. It worked once upon a time. This is once upon a very critical *now*. "If you feel strongly that the human race is worth saving, we have to eliminate animal agriculture," says ex-cattleman Howard Lyman, author of *Mad Cowboy*. "The grassroots is the only way this fight will be won."

Although averting climatic disaster would seem to be sufficient motivation for a dietary rethink, animal agriculture is also responsible, in part or in huge part, for the majority of other ecological plagues we face: water shortages; habitat destruction; impaired air quality; deforestation, including the loss of the rain forests said to be "the lungs of the earth"; overfishing (our oceans are so imperiled that *any* fishing in the twenty-first century is overfishing); ocean dumping; acid rain; and even the energy crisis because the energy demands of Big Agra are so great.

In addition, the estimates are that anywhere from 30 to an astounding 45 percent of our planet's landmass (that's from the International Livestock Research Institute) is devoted to either grazing or growing feed crops for livestock. This is a shameful waste of resources. Devoting vast acreage to monoculture, raising a single crop such as corn for animal feed, is no friend of topsoil, and overgrazing erodes topsoil like nobody's business. University of Sydney professor John Crawford estimates that we have about sixty years of topsoil left. That may not mean much to us urban dwellers, but topsoil is the layer that allows plants to grow. No topsoil, no food—for anybody.

Then there's the pollution piece. The National Resources Defense Council cites that pollution from waste "lagoons" and manure "sprayfields"—Don Draper himself couldn't have come up with better spin terms—are threats to human health. Producing sufficient pork and other animal products for current world demand requires raising animals in numbers that only factory farms, those CAFOs we talked about earlier, can produce. A staggering amount of air and water pollution is one result. (The documentary film *Speciesism: The Movie* illustrates the effects of this pollution on people in rural North Carolina, a major pork-producing area, in a way you'll never forget.)

Earth Day Every Day

While some giants of the environmental movement have come to see that *living green* starts with *eating green*, even the most cursory search reveals that many well-known environmentalists and most of the large environmental organizations are oblivious to this issue. Another compelling documentary, *Cowspiracy*, attempts to discover why these watchdog groups aren't watching very well.

Solving our ecological problems with smaller cars and smaller farms is a comforting fantasy—the way I sometimes fantasized in my single-mom days that marrying a movie star or becoming Oprah's favorite author would rescue my daughter and me from all our struggles. But those daydreams, however remote, were *possible*. Sustainably feeding a human population of 7 billion and growing simply cannot happen without a major shift toward plant-based eating.

In the United States, this shift has been happening, slowly but steadily, since 2007; in 2013, a full 500,000,000 fewer animals—half a whopping billion!—were slaughtered than would have been at previous consumption levels. Even so, Americans still eat more meat than almost anyone else, and the unfortunate global trend is toward greater meat and dairy consumption than ever before in history, fueled by a massive and relatively recent appetite for meat in China and India.

So, we're back to hopeless, right? I can't tell some person halfway around the world what to eat. But you know what? We do influence others, even those we don't know, and we do it more in this Internet era than ever before. You or I can post a link to a tasty Good Karma recipe on a social media site, and as it gets shared and shared some more, somebody just might prepare a vegan dinner in Hangzhou or Mumbai. That's one dinner to the good. I realize that none of us, alone, can save the world, but all of us together can. In fact, we have to. There's no one else to do it.

Jim's Good Karma Story

About a dozen years ago, I became curious about the optimal diet for humans. I had no medical issues. I wasn't fat. Just curious. So I began with a search for the author of a health book that I'd read a dozen years earlier. When I found his new book, Amazon suggested three others for me to consider. One thing led to another, and after reading thirty or forty books, I concluded that a whole-food, plant-based (WFPB) diet was optimal for human health.

Then I read two more books that focused on how our food choices affect the environment, world hunger, and the suffering of animals. Suddenly, I had what I called my "blinding flash of the obvious," and said to myself, "Oh my God, we're eating the wrong food!"

Having learned that most chronic disease could be easily prevented or even reversed with an optimal diet, I decided to leverage my consulting and executive background—I'd been an executive vice president at Ralph Lauren—to assist corporations in lowering their out-of-control health care costs. Although that particular endeavor has yet to bear much fruit, many others have.

During the past ten years, I have made it my business to get to know the leaders of the plant-based movement. And when my book, *Healthy Eating, Healthy World*, was published, the three most celebrated experts in the plant-based world—Drs. T. Colin Campbell, Caldwell Esselstyn Jr., and Dean Ornish—provided endorsements. Shortly thereafter I was invited to join the board of directors of the T. Colin Campbell Center for Nutrition Studies.

There's more. I've become a prolific blogger, posting some thousand articles on my site, hpjmh.com. And as the book and blog picked up steam, I began to get paid speaking engagements and opportunities to meet with powerful world leaders, including film director James Cameron and media titan Ted Turner. When well-known leaders start making enough noise, more people will learn what we must do to preserve Mother Nature's ability to sustain us as a species. What could be more important than that?

Last but not least, I'm part of a small group that launched The Plantrician Project (plantrician.org), a not-for-profit organization with a powerful mission: to educate, equip, and empower medical practitioners to embrace true "health reform" by promoting health instead of just managing disease. Our aim is to bring back the ancient wisdom of Hippocrates, "Let food be thy medicine and medicine be thy food."

My new way of eating has exceeded my wildest dreams. I have found my definite purpose in life, launched a brand-new career, and have never been happier. And there's a bonus. I mentioned earlier that I wasn't sick or fat before changing my diet, but maybe I was sicker than I thought. Within a year of shifting to the WFPB diet, I lost twenty pounds, got sick less often, slept much better, and noticed an improvement in my performance in the bedroom—to name just a few benefits.

—**J. Morris Hicks**, speaker, blogger, and author of
Healthy Eating, Healthy World. hpjmh.com

18

......

Food and Health and
Price and Justice

On the first Saturday that felt like summer, William and I put Forbes in his doggie stroller and took the subway to Union Square, site of the biggest farmers' market in New York City. It's a carnival atmosphere, with mouthwatering produce and fresh flowers and prepared foods from somebody's actual kitchen.

While I gawked at everything, William had a plan: tomatoes, real ones whose roots were in dirt, available for only a few months of the year, but during those months, they taste like the ones his mother grew in her garden. He spotted an organic booth with some attractive specimens and put six of them, medium-sized, in a bag. "That'll be $23.50," the farmer said, and William, stunned into submission, pulled out a twenty and a five and paid the guy. I was standing nearby about to purchase a bell pepper, but I put it back, figuring we'd just shot half the budget on six tomatoes.

Now, they turned out to be splendid tomatoes. We savored them, one each for three days, and joked about how tomatoes were ranking on the NASDAQ. We could do that because we can afford, from time to time anyway, to unexpectedly part with $23.50. There's no way to look at food and karma, however, without thinking of people for whom $23.50 is supposed to feed a family for a day—or for a week. There's a lot going on here: the personal issue of feeding our families well on the money we have, the local issue of people in our own cities and towns who deny themselves nutritious foods because of the cost, and the global issue that malnutrition plays a role in the deaths of some five million children every year—80 percent of those in countries where feed crops are grown for doomed livestock.

Third World hunger is recognizable in emaciated frames and swollen bellies. American hunger is often masked by the obesity that derives from a surfeit of cheap calories coupled with a chronic lack of nutrition. This is a complex situation, touching on fields beyond my expertise—politics and policy, economics, public health, even the way a society chooses to define human rights. So I consulted experts. One of these, Jill Nussinow, MS, RD (TheVeggieQueen.com), is a champion of local farmers and the foods they midwife into being. "I want to hand my money to the people who grew the food," she says. "I'd rather have one perfect tomato, one tomato grown with love, than six from the grocery store that won't do anything for me."

GKT

While promoters of genetically modified organisms want to add to this list, foods that are most often genetically modified as of this writing are soybeans and their products, canola and cottonseed oils, sugar from sugar beets, corn, and Hawaiian papaya. Because farmed animals, even fish, are fed corn, factor this in if you still eat some animal products.

Although trained in science, Nussinow also has a sense of the subtle energies of foods fresh from the earth. "I was away on business and missed our farmers' market days," she recounted, "so I went to a supermarket and bought romaine hearts in a bag and made my husband a salad. He said, 'Where did you get this lettuce? It's completely lifeless.' Now, my husband isn't somebody who gives a lot of thought to food, but he noticed the difference, even though this was organic romaine grown in California where we live, so it hadn't come from across the country. It was just missing something."

Hearing her story brought to mind one of my own. As a child, I thought fruit was pointless and that people who put apples in trick-or-treat bags had something against kids. But one summer, the blessing inside the trauma of my parents' divorce and my mom's marrying an air force captain and moving to Europe was finding myself on a Mediterranean beach—Nice, France, to be exact. We didn't have beaches in Kansas City, but in this place far away, bright blue sky met deep blue water, and vendors selling fruits of every color lined the walkways. We bought a mixed basket; I chose a pear and took a bite. Instantly, catechism class made sense: Eve had sold us all up the river so she could have a piece of fruit. It must have been this fruit! If it was, I thought guiltily, I'd have done the same thing.

For the rest of the week, we ate pears. There may have been dinners in the imposing stone hotel, but all I remember are the pears: sweet, juicy, ripened on trees so I was eating something finished. Every piece of fruit I'd had in my eleven years until then had been snatched early from the tree or vine. It was incomplete, the way the *Mona Lisa* we'd seen in the Louvre just days before would have been incomplete without her eyes or her smile or her oddly crossed hands.

Whether or not to use honey has always been left to personal conscience among vegans. The majority of modern vegans avoid it. Those who use it look for honey from ethical bee-keepers who don't truck their bees hither and yon to pollinate crops, and who harvest the honey in springtime after the bees have had their fill. For more on bees, see the documentary *Queen of the Sun* (QueenoftheSun.com).

The Economics of Animals and Vegetables

But if all this great food falls off trees and pushes up from the soil, why is the price so high? I asked David Robinson Simon, JD, author of *Meatonomics: How the Rigged Economics of Meat and Dairy Make You Consume Too Much*, to make sense of the nonsensical. To give you the full benefit of what he had to say, here's a somewhat abridged transcript of that interview:

VM: Why is produce expensive?

DS: *Produce does seem expensive, but only when compared to animal foods. Produce is not heavily subsidized, and the industry externalizes far fewer of its costs on society. An externalized cost is a cost that parties to a transaction do not bear but instead impose on third parties, like if I were to throw my garbage into a park instead of paying a garbage service to collect it. Externalized costs of animal food production include, among other things, its contribution to climate change, water pollution, and health consequences such as coronary heart disease.*

VM: But why do organic fruits and vegetables cost even more? And why are local, organic products—in my locale, anyway—off the charts?

DS: *Organic inputs like fertilizer are more expensive than inorganic. Also, the absence of chemicals in organic produce means that more labor is required to perform tasks that chemicals would do otherwise, such as pulling weeds. And local produce is typically grown on relatively small farms that lack the economies of scale enjoyed by larger agribusinesses.*

VM: But historically, wasn't it meat that cost a lot? What happened?

DS: *In the past few years, meat prices have been rising steadily, but they're still much lower than they should be. The retail price of meat should be roughly three times higher than it is; a $5 Big Mac should really cost $13. The artificially low prices reflect heavy government subsidies and externalization of costs on a massive scale. To put these costs in perspective, roughly $251 billion worth of animal foods are sold each year in the United States, and in the course of generating these sales, the industry externalizes roughly $414 billion of costs (or about $1.70 of externalized costs per $1 of retail sales).*

VM: What happens when we look beyond the United States? Do our food choices really matter in terms of being good global citizens?

DS: *Yes, in many ways. Americans consume more meat per capita than anyone else on the planet (except the tiny and statistically insignificant Luxembourg). That means we externalize our costs on the rest of the planet in disproportionate ways—climate change, for example, and the many negative effects that climate change has on farming in developing countries, like water loss, erosion, desertification, and other problems that make it hard to grow food.*

VM: I remember when people were going vegetarian en masse as a result of reading *Diet for a Small Planet* and believing that if we stopped eating meat, it would end world hunger. Is the theoretical feed-those-crops-to-humans-instead-of-livestock argument relevant in any practical way?

DS: *Ecologist David Pimentel said that if all the grain fed to livestock in the United States were instead fed to people, 800 million additional people could be fed. That's because it takes six pounds of plant-based protein to raise one pound of animal-based protein. Whether a switch like this could be achieved logistically is a great question, but the 6:1 ratio is an important equation that should make us think about and refocus our priorities.*

Dollars and Sense

This helps me—and I hope you, too—see that there's a lot to "economies of scale," applying not only to fresh foods, but to minimally processed products from tiny companies as well. The woman in Idaho making organic sprouted nut butters in a rented kitchen doesn't have the same fiscal advantages as one of the peanut butter companies that's a household name, but she's able to get the nutrition and life force of fresh food into a jar. She can't give you cheap, but she will give you value—which is all well and good, unless you simply can't afford it.

The government subsidies that have kept at least some meat products affordable have also helped the retail price of mass-produced processed foods go down by some 40 percent since 1980—precisely the same amount that the cost of fruits and vegetables has risen in that same time period. Despite all this, it is fully possible to eat as a healthy vegan on a budget, even a tight one, but it does call for some reeducation, and a willingness to cook from scratch, something many people don't believe they have time for, or simply don't know how to do. Raw food, of all styles of plant-based eating, has been criticized most for being pricey, even elitist. My friend Elizabeth in Kansas City, a home ec major who loves to try out different cuisines, looked into this one and afterward deadpanned, "I made a raw pie. It cost $37."

No doubt about it, organic nuts, coconut, dates, berries, and tropical fruits don't come cheap. In addition, a raw fooder who requires fresh produce every day can never follow the classic budgeting advice to periodically "go a week without groceries," turning instead to whatever grains, dried beans, and frozen and canned goods are on hand. But raw or not, we're all supposed to be eating fresh produce daily, and raw-food families figure out how to do this affordably, the way any of us with enough means to make choices figure out how to do the things we value and prioritize. To eat extraordinary food without winning the lottery, consider these suggestions:

- At any income level, you can follow the basics of kitchen economics: eat at home more often, prepare more meals from basic ingredients (vegetables, grains, beans) instead of from packages, and stop paying for convenience—prewashed greens and prechopped onions are nice, but there is a cost.

- Produce in season, wherever you buy it, will be both fresher and cheaper. And don't judge by appearances. Cosmetically imperfect fruit—i.e., apples in bags with a bruise here and there—can be just as tasty and health-promoting as those sold singly, and the difference in price can allow you to buy more food, or upgrade to organic.

- Superfoods shouldn't be reserved for the super-rich. Don't be fooled by some big-ticket fruit, berry, seed, juice, or powder that comes from somewhere exotic, costs a mint, and will supposedly cure everything from crow's-feet to spider veins. A superfood is nothing but an edible plant that comes in a color. This means fruits, vegetables, beans, seeds, spices, herbs, and tea (green and white tea, in particular). They're in every grocery store, and if you have some soil and sun, you can grow herbs and vegetables yourself.

- A yard with no garden is like a home with no love. Plant something. Zucchini practically grows itself, and kale is so hearty you can keep harvesting it after a frost. No yard? Remember sprouts and microgreens (chapter 5). And herbs such as bay leaves, chervil, dill, mint, and parsley will grow in pots on a sunny windowsill.

- Even if you're eating high-raw, you can take advantage of the fill-up factor of some cooked foods, i.e., root vegetables, whole grains, and legumes, some of the lowest-priced foods in the marketplace. Conversely, eating greens and other water-rich vegetables raw is highly cost effective. Half a pound of raw spinach makes a nice salad for two; half a pound of spinach after it's cooked is a side dish for one.

- Consolidate your buying power by joining with others in a food co-op or CSA (Community Supported Agriculture). In a storefront co-op, you can work a few hours a month in return for discounted groceries; or become part of a private co-op where you and your fellow members can order in case lots, wholesale, just as if you were a small store. With a CSA, you buy a share in an organic farm for the season, saving big on produce and learning about vegetables (sometimes fruits, too) that may be new to you.

- When shopping more conventionally, some stores are just cheaper than others, even for organic items. Unless you find that they're underpaying their workers or cutting corners in some other offensive ways, go where you get the most for your money.

- Shop the bulk bins at your natural food store for its lowest prices on nuts, seeds, legumes, grains, and dried fruits.

- See what choices, prices, and quality you find shopping Internet retailers. The cost is sometimes low enough to cover the shipping.

- "When you're at the farmers' market, talk with the people behind the tables, usually the farmers and their families," says Jill Nussinow. "Ask if they have any seconds, produce that doesn't look perfect so they're not displaying it, but that they might be willing to sell at a substantial discount." Another tip is to go to the market in the hour before closing. Farmers prefer to go home with an empty truck, so many are selling what's left at a fraction of the price they were asking earlier. And if you have an EBT card, you can use it at farmers' markets in many areas.

- Get an online education in plant-based penny-pinching. There's Ellen Jaffe Jones's popular Facebook page, Eat Vegan on 4 Dollars a Day, based on her best-selling book of the same title; and Lisa Viger's blog *Raw on $10 a Day*

(RawOn10.com—yes, $10 is more than $4 but developing superpowers does have value).

- Those of us with discretionary income may need to be willing to spend more on groceries. It won't be that much more, since you're saving on the animal foods and junk foods you no longer eat—and being in good health saves money, too. For example, if you pay for your own medical insurance and you're healthy enough to buy a high-deductible plan, you can save $1,000 a year or more—and you may qualify for a health savings account (HSA), deductible from your federal income tax.

- Become invested in ending hunger, domestically or globally. If you're serious about this karma thing, you get it that "We're all connected" isn't just something from a guided meditation with Celtic flutes in the background. As long as one child is hungry anywhere on this earth, I can't be fully nourished, in a holistic way, because that child I'll never know is, at some level, a part of me, and of you. So let's do something. It's laudable to volunteer at a soup kitchen (it doesn't have be Christmas or Thanksgiving), and to support the work of organizations feeding the hungry around the world with plant-based foods. These include A Well-Fed World (AWellFedWorld.org), Food for Life Global (ffl.org/en), and VegFam (VegFamCharity.org/uk). In addition, learn about the issues affecting people closer to home. David Simon's *Meatonomics* is one great book; *Stuffed and Starved*, by Raj Patel, and *Food Politics*, by Marion Nestle, are others. Armed with information, you can lend your vote and your voice to a just food system.

Bottom line on bottom lines: treat yourself well and share generously with others.

Be smart with your money and smarter with your health. Elect public officials who see hunger as unacceptable. Support the individuals and businesses that are helping create a humane and sustainable world. And make choices every day that will bring that world into being.

19

......

But Everybody Says
Something Different

You may at this point be thinking, "I want good karma. I want to save animals and feel happy and look good when I'm seventy, but I'm confused about food and nutrition: everybody says something different." I hear you. And I hear *them*—the countless conflicting voices with views on food and nutrition that don't just differ on technicalities, but can seem to be all over the map. Sometimes I think the wisest response to all the he said/she said is to go deep inside, get really still, and allow for your own truth to surface. What resonates with you? What makes sense? Envision yourself a year from now, and ten years from now, if you continue eating and living precisely as you have been. No changes. Just keep on keepin' on, and a year from now, and ten years from now, what does your body look like? What does your life look like? How has the way you've lived for this projected decade shaped the lives of others and the direction of our culture?

Next, do the same visualization, inserting some way of eating you've considered—paleo or Mediterranean or farm-to-table omnivore or something else. In one year, and in ten, what does your body look like? And your life? And what about the lives of those you've influenced and impacted, the amount of suffering you've curtailed, the contribution you've made to what a spiritual teacher of mine used to call "the upward progression of the universe"?

Now envision that you've made the Good Karma choice. You're eating exclusively from the plant kingdom with lots of fresh, raw foods the colors of spring bouquets and Christmas windows. You allow yourself some leeway in your food choices for when life intervenes, but for the most part you're eating whole, unprocessed vegetables, fruits, legumes, nuts, seeds, and whole grains the way nature presents them, the best food you can afford prepared in the best ways you know how—usually simple and basic, sometimes epicurean and out of this world. After a year, what does your body look like? And after ten years? After a year and after ten, what does your life look like? And after a year and after a decade, how has the way you've lived affected other people, other animals, and the evolutionary trajectory of life on earth?

GKT

Visit the website of a sanctuary for farmed animals—find a comprehensive list of them at sanctuaries.org. Read the animals' stories and look into their eyes. Become the adoptive human of some enchanting pig, cow, turkey, chicken, duck, goose, goat, sheep, or rabbit. And if you can visit in person, OMG—your life will change in such a good way.

When I do that exercise, the Good Karma Diet comes out hands down as the way to health and fulfillment. It's also delicious! I wondered for twenty years why that wasn't just the end of the story. In terms of how to feed ourselves, we've found the pot of gold at the end of the rainbow. Why not check that off our species-wide bucket list and move on to world peace? But not everybody sees it this way, and the nutritional landscape is polarized as never before.

There are experts who sing the praises of a Mediterranean diet, complete with olive oil, and others who are adamant that those studies were flawed and that extracted oil of any sort damages the endothelial cells lining our blood vessels, increasing our chances of a heart attack. *(What I do: get most of my fat from seeds and nuts, but there is olive oil in my pantry to use in a vinaigrette dressing or to sauté an onion.)*

If the pundits weren't so civilized, they'd come to fisticuffs over soy. One faction claims it's the wonder bean and a cure-all. The other says that soy-eating women develop breast cancer and soy-eating men develop breasts. *(What I do: read the actual studies. They're not all that intimidating, and what they say, to an overwhelming extent, is that soy, like all legumes, is a really good food. Its phyto [plant] estrogens, rather than leading to cancer formation, early puberty, or feminization of males, actually protect against these. They do this by attaching to the receptors where xeno [foreign] estrogens, from plastics and pesticides, could otherwise attach and cause trouble. Unless you're allergic to it, soy, especially in the form of fresh beans [edamame], tempeh, and miso, is a positive addition to the diet. Tofu and soy foods with the taste and texture of meat, milk, and other familiar fare can be helpful, too. In a Good Karma Diet with more raw food, you won't consume as much soy as somebody taking a different tack on being vegan might, but what you do eat should be just fine.)*

Some experts espouse a vegan, near-vegan, or raw vegan diet; others, a raw diet that isn't vegan. *(What I do: vegan, about 70 percent raw.)* Among the raw folks, we find recommendations for a very high amount of fruit in the diet and very little fat, and also recommendations for restricting fruit intake. *(What I do: I eat fruit but rarely by itself. My blood sugar likes it when I have fruit with oatmeal or muesli, or raw granola, or unsweetened soy yogurt, or some nuts.)* And of course, there are some legitimate and some more, shall we say, *independent* authorities who oppose any iteration of vegetarianism. *(What I do: disagree with them. That's allowed.)*

With this dizzying array of sparring opinions, it's no wonder some people say, "It's too much: just give me the Killer Burger and a couple of prescriptions." Part of prudence is to weigh conflicting opinions against your own good judgment and your instinctive inklings. Other than for research purposes, I don't seek out the books or websites of people who have an entirely different dietary worldview. I know how I want to live, and I look for the physicians, nutritionists, and authors who can help me do it best.

The Great Divide

Of all the differences of opinion, one stands out. I call it The Great Divide. In popular books and on PBS specials, we see, on the one hand, support for a diet that consists either entirely or primarily of whole plant foods. On the other, we see a distrust of carbohydrates, and a recommendation of some variation on the "meat and greens" theme: a high-protein, high-fat, very low carbohydrate diet of flesh, eggs, nuts and seeds, non-starchy vegetables, and the lowest-sugar fruits. Unless we're talking pure paleo, experts in this camp probably approve of fat-reduced dairy products. Many are also good with varying amounts of legumes and whole grains, although some are so anti-carb that they have a problem with even unsweetened, cholesterol-lowering steel-cut oats.

Still, there are points at which these disparate points of view intersect. All agree:

- The foods that benefit us come from nature; manufactured foods, especially when consumed in excess or to the exclusion of natural foods, are harmful.

- Whole foods, without parts missing and molecules deranged, are the gold standard.

- Refined sugar and high-fructose corn syrup are killers, and although probably not harmful to healthy people in small amounts, no concentrated sweetener—maple syrup, agave nectar, etc.—can be said to actually benefit the body.

Well, that's a start, and enough of one to find common ground. Nobody is saying that sweets and refined flour products—cotton candy and sugary cereal and bread so soft and white we used to smash it to play Holy Communion back in Catholic school—are the way to go. The primary point of contention has to do with complex carbohydrates—those found in vegetables, beans, and whole grains— and the sugar that's in fresh fruit. Are these naturally occurring carbohydrates important foods for humans, or just "carbs" to be avoided?

In Defense of a Macronutrient

Neal Barnard, MD, president of Physicians Committee for Responsible Medicine (PCRM) and author of *Dr. Neal Barnard's Program for Reversing Diabetes*, takes up the case for carbs: "Carbohydrates are the natural fuel for the body. Just as your car runs on gasoline, your brain, muscles, and all the rest of you run on glucose, the natural sugar that is provided by carbohydrate." In PCRM's research studies, plant-based diets were used for weight problems and diabetes. The findings were that when people got away from meats, cheese, etc., and increased their intake of carbohydrate-rich whole grains, vegetables, fruits, and beans, weight loss occurred consistently, along with decreased abdominal fat and improved blood pressure, cholesterol, and triglyceride levels.

The crux of the matter, then, seems to be the difference between a refined sugar—soda, candy, pastries—or a refined starch—polished white rice, instant mashed potatoes, a white-flour hamburger bun— and a complex carbohydrate. This is a grain, bean, or vegetable, presenting as a complete package that includes protein, fiber, and a little fat. Metabolized as a whole food, this is something that the body— including a body that's been ill-fed, overfed, and sugar-fed—can understand and deal with. Even the sugar in fresh fruit is slowed down in the metabolic ballet by the fiber and small amounts of protein and fat these foods in their natural state contain. In other words, nature got it right. Imagine that.

GKT

Licorice tea, and herbal blends based on licorice, can be a real help in kicking a sugar habit. Licorice tastes sweet without sugar, and it causes cortisol and other adrenal hormones to break down more slowly, allowing them to be more available for blood sugar stabilization.

Do some people have to be more careful about sugar than others? Yes. Some of us have become sugar-sensitive. Having your blood sugar tested by your doctor is one way to determine this, but feeling spacey or dizzy or headachy after a rich dessert, or even a glass of fruit juice on an empty stomach, tells you a lot. If you're sugar-sensitive, you need to assiduously avoid refined sugars and refined starches. Even whole-grain flour is more refined than the whole, unground grain from which that flour came; if you're sugar-sensitive, you'll notice the difference. The sugar-sensitive need to exercise caution around dried fruits and sweet desserts, even when these contain no refined sugars, and high-glycemic white potatoes.

But the plant kingdom is vast; even when avoiding these relatively few foods, you can still eat widely and well. And if you feel that consuming a little more protein and a little less carbohydrate than some other vegans do works better for you, do that. "There are all kinds of dietary patterns that protect health," says Virginia Messina, MPH, RD, coauthor of *Vegan for Her*, "but they all seem to have the underlying theme of lots of whole plant foods and minimal processed foods. I don't think there is much evidence that cutting carbs drastically is a good or necessary thing. But, some people may do a little bit better by replacing some carbs with protein and fat from plant sources."

Is Meat Really Bad for People, or Do You Just like Animals?

After William and I watched *Fed Up*, a well-crafted documentary about the evils of sugar and processed foods, he said to me: "I think I get it now: it's the sugar that's bad for your health; not eating meat, eggs, and dairy is an ethical thing." My heart sank—not so much that this was his conclusion (I happen to know he lives with someone who can set him straight) but that this was probably the conclusion of a lot of people who saw that film. And this brings us to the second point that separates the plant-based experts from the meat-based experts: whether or not any actual, physiological harm comes from eating animal foods.

"There is no question," says Dr. Barnard, "that animal products raise the risk of weight problems, diabetes, high blood pressure, heart disease, and certain cancers." They also cause inflammation, a factor in virtually every degenerative disease, while any accounting of anti-inflammatory foods looks like a shopping list for the produce market: berries, cherries, cruciferous vegetables, leafy greens, papaya, pineapple, sweet potatoes, and nuts and seeds.

Meat has cholesterol and the saturated fat from which the body makes more cholesterol. The salmon we're routinely told to consume in abundance has, according to the USDA, as much cholesterol as hamburger. Dairy products are the primary source of saturated fat in the American diet, and when the fat in them is reduced or removed, the relative protein content goes up. This may sound good, but the work of Dr. T. Colin Campbell of the China Study and other researchers around the world has shown convincingly that excess *animal* protein is harmful, even promoting the growth of cancer cells, while plant protein, in virtually any amount, appears to have no ill effects. Animal foods lack fiber and vitamin C, and when it comes to disease-fighting antioxidants, they can't compete with a limp carrot.

Joel Kahn, MD, holistic cardiologist, Wayne State Medical School professor, and author of *The Whole Heart Solution*, wrote a fascinating article for MindBodyGreen.com about some of the less often discussed problems of flesh foods in the human diet. These include:

- Insulin-like Growth Factor 1 (IGF-1) is linked to breast and prostate cancers, and levels are consistently higher in people who eat meat.

- Low levels of methionine, an amino acid found largely in animal products, correlate with longer life spans.

- A Cleveland Clinic study found that meat eaters produce a metabolite called Trimethylamine-N-oxide (TMAO) that promotes atherosclerosis and heart disease.

- Persistent Organic Pollutants (POPs) are synthetic chemicals including dioxins, DDT, and PCBs. These accumulate in fat, and we consume them when we eat foods such as meat, butter, and fish.

- Advanced glycation end products (AGEs) occur naturally in many foods, more in meats than in plant foods, and when the meat is grilled, the levels go up. Curiously, AGEs lead to accelerated *aging*, and are associated with brain inflammation, diabetes, heart disease, and cancer.

With all this known, why do we hear only about what's wrong with cake and cola and so seldom, in the mainstream media anyway, about problems with animal foods? I think it's because saltine crackers and cookie dough have no redeeming nutritional qualities, while animal products have some. These have been overemphasized by powerful industries making it easy to demonize sweets and give meat, fish, eggs, and dairy a pass. Meat has protein and red meat has iron; cow's milk has calcium; salmon has omega-3 fatty acids. And Jack the Ripper may have had a charming personality, but there are other factors at play.

The heart of the matter is that animal foods carry cultural currency. They're rich, and people like them. They're associated with masculinity, even though the same saturated fat that clogs arteries to the heart, leading to a coronary, clogs arteries to the penis, leading to "That's all right, darling, it happens to everybody sometimes." These foods are believed to build strength; yet the strongest animals on earth are vegetarian, and the strongest man on earth, as I write this, is Patrik Baboumian, a vegan living in Germany. Animal foods are aligned, in the United States, anyway, with patriotism and family values, but the health care crisis they've helped bring about could bankrupt the country. And families are devastated when loved ones succumb to the diseases wrought by the Standard American Diet (SAD), with way too many animal foods *and* way too many refined and processed starches and sugars.

Perhaps animal foods get two thumbs up from some popular experts because they believe that getting people to cut out, or even cut down on, sugary, salty manufactured foods is a tall enough order. Adding meat and dairy to the list would be too much to give up. They don't understand that once the "aha!" moment about eating animals happens, it's no longer a matter of giving up.

Those health practitioners urging us to adopt a plant-based diet point to findings that repeatedly show vegans as leaner than their omnivorous and lacto-ovo-vegetarian peers, with healthier cholesterol, blood pressure, and blood glucose levels. To join their ranks, I share this straightforward prescription from Houston bariatric specialist Garth Davis, MD: "Stop loading up on excess protein. Stop eating diseased, tortured animals that cause inflammation. Stop fearing real carbs that have fed thriving populations for all of civilization. Feast on beautiful, delicious fruits and vegetables. Eat food that looks alive. Eat food that has been grown and made with love."

Opponents will argue that any carb is a bad carb, or that "certain people" require animal foods for various mysterious reasons, or that plant eaters can become deficient in vitamin B_{12}, or iron, or calcium. So can omnivores, for that matter, but here's my point: Despite the nutritional bickering we read about and see on TV, the science is overwhelming in its support of whole plant foods. And Kaiser Permanente, America's largest managed care consortium, an entity with a serious economic stake in its members' staying healthy, published the following in its peer-reviewed journal: "Healthy eating may be best achieved with a plant-based diet, which we define as a regimen that encourages whole, plant-based foods and discourages meats, dairy products, and eggs as well as all refined and processed foods. . . . Physicians should consider recommending a plant-based diet to all their patients, especially those with high blood pressure, diabetes, cardiovascular disease, or obesity."

And if that's not enough, remember: as important as health is, there's more to this. It's also about healing a planet, and responding to a prompting of the soul. It's about hearing the prayers of suffering animals, however it is they pray, and responding to those prayers like a guardian angel.

20

......

Gimme a V!

t may be nerdy, but I'm really fond of acronyms. They make charming little packages that belie the amount of wisdom within them. When I talk about going veg, I turn "vegan" into an acronym that stands for:

- Validate your choice,

- Embody a healthy lifestyle,

- Get to know other Good Karma diners,

- Add more to your life than you subtract, and

- Never forget the animals.

You may have already ascertained that I *like* the word "vegan." Not everybody does, and most of those who don't are vegans! Or, they eat as vegans but have reservations about identifying as such. In some cases, it's because a person doesn't want to commit. They may eat a virtually plant-exclusive diet but want some wiggle room that they believe coming out as a vegan would preclude.

In other cases, folks don't want to be confused with "animal rights people," although I think that being aligned with any valid liberation movement is a compliment.

There are also people deeply invested in the health aspects of this way of eating who prefer nomenclature other than the v-word. They don't want to be classed with "cupcake vegans," people who avoid animal products but delight in every veganized recreational food a clever cook or company can develop.

We used to have an easy answer: two terms. "Ethical vegan" was the descriptor for someone concerned about animal cruelty and who refused not only animal foods but also fur and leather, animal-exploiting entertainment (rodeos, bullfights, circuses), and animal-tested toiletries and household products (we'll get to these in chapter 23). "Health vegan" applied to those who stayed away from animal products and other foods they considered less than ideal; coats and cosmetics didn't enter in. For whatever reason—and perhaps it's simply because so many of us nowadays think of ourselves as ethical/health/environmental vegans—the old phrases have fallen out of favor and people who want to avoid "vegan" call themselves "plant-based," "plant-strong," or even "better than vegan."

I champion the traditional word, however, because people know what it means. I remember when they didn't. They'd ask if *vegan* had something to do with the planet where Spock on *Star Trek* came from. I feel that tossing out seventy-plus years of educating the populace is highly inefficient. Therefore, you're getting an acronym for V-E-G-A-N. If you don't care for the word, you can still get something out of the explanations.

V: Validate Your Choice

This means learning what you need to learn to take the Good Karma path successfully for yourself and, if applicable, for your family, and also to answer the questions others are bound to have about what you're doing. Is it fair that you'll be called upon to explain yourself when there are people eating fast food every day and giving their toddlers bottles filled with Kool-Aid? Of course it isn't, but vegans are a voluntary minority: different, quaint, fascinating, admirable in some ways, perhaps, but still a bit suspect.

People will want to know where you get your protein. "Where do you think I get it?" is the response Marty Davey, MS, RD (LaDivaDietitian.com), likes to use, claiming that the person who asks the question owns the conversation. If you're upright and not hospitalized, the questioner is going to have to concede that you obviously get this vital macronutrient *somewhere*, bringing them, perhaps for the first time, to the realization that "protein" is not a synonym for "meat."

They'll sometimes ask about other nutrients, too, so go over chapter 14, "Letters and Numbers and Science, Oh My!," until you have those fundamentals down. In addition to basic nutrition questions, you'll be asked about animal issues and about opposing dietary views. For example: "Weren't animals put here for us to eat?" *Funny, we don't think we're here for sharks to eat. But seriously: we can be healthy—healthier, in fact—without killing and eating animals, so let's give them a break.*

"If we didn't eat them, wouldn't animals overtake the earth?" *No, because we intentionally breed them. Moreover, from an environmental perspective—the methane, the manure lagoons, the deforestation— they've taken over already, through no fault of their own.*

"But shouldn't we eat like Paleolithic man, mostly lean meat with a few berries and leaves and nuts?" *That's somewhat turned around. According to the best archaeology, our Paleolithic predecessors weren't so much hunter-gatherers as gatherer-hunters. Humans have never been equipped for a kill the way a tiger or a jackal is; our ancestors ate some meat, yes, but fossil evidence reveals that they also ate a huge amount of plant material.*

It can be overwhelming to think that you'll be called upon to be a fount of information about something you've just discovered yourself. Saying, "I really don't know, but I'll look into that" is always a reasonable response, although reading this book and two or three others (see Appendix B) should give you enough of a foundation to discuss these matters intelligently, whether at a family reunion or on national TV.

E: Embody a Healthy Lifestyle

Whatever your reason for going vegan, people will form their opinion of it based on how you look and behave. You do not have to become an athlete (although doing so is a great coup for the cause) or come up with a body so beautiful you volunteer for PETA's "I'd rather go naked than wear fur" campaign. You just have to look at least as well as you ever did, and preferably a little better. If you're following Good Karma principles, this will happen with no further effort on your part. The green smoothies, the salads, the berries, all the rainbow cuisine that will make up your daily diet beautify from the inside out.

GKT

Stand more than you sit. It's been shown that men who sit the most—even if they exercise regularly—develop heart failure more often than those who stand several hours a day. Joel Kahn, MD, author of *The Holistic Heart Book*, says, "Sitting is the new smoking."

Health is more than nutrition, though. You need to get enough sleep or you'll look haggard and worn, green smoothies notwithstanding. If you smoke, stop: cigarettes will give you wrinkles before they give you cancer, and that doesn't help any animals. You need to exercise because all that oxygen and increased circulation will show on your face—and having some muscle tone won't hurt, either.

Be sure there's fun in your life every day because happy is even rarer than ripped, and if your life looks like one worth aspiring toward, you'll inspire others to that aspiration. And be kind to humans, too, even the annoying ones.

G: Get to Know Other Good Karma Diners

Billy James Cobin, creative director at a New York political consulting company, has said: "Emotion trumps logic. Tribe trumps everything." I remember the spot where I was standing when I heard this. For me, this answered the riddle of the ex-vegan. People have emotional connections to food that can draw them back to old habits, but "tribe trumps everything." With other people in your life doing this, too, you're golden. You need your peeps. We all do.

Find us on Facebook and Twitter, and check out our YouTube channels and bountiful blogs. BonzaiAphrodite.com, VeggieGirl.com, ChoosingRaw.com, JLGoesVegan.com, RevelinginRaw.com, and SavetheKales.com are a handful of the hundreds of informative and entertaining veggie blogs out there. Even I have one—Main StreetVegan.net/blog—which includes a new post every Tuesday; I contribute the first of the month, while bright and thoughtful graduates of Main Street Vegan Academy post the other weeks.

You can meet vegetarians, vegans, and the veg-curious in three dimensions, too. We're at the gym and yoga class (wear a vegan T-shirt so kindred spirits will know you're there). We're shopping at the natural foods store (look at what people are buying and start a conversation). We're also at festivals in large and small cities across North America and around the world. Some of these are huge and long-standing—Toronto, Boston, Portland (the Portland that's out West), and London (the London that has Big Ben)—and others are total delights in surprising places: Bethlehem, Pennsylvania; Rehoboth Beach, Delaware; St. Catharine's, Ontario.

There are also conferences. Physicians Committee for Responsible Medicine hosts seminars about plant-based nutrition that are so medically official that health care professionals receive continuing education credits for attending. For sheer summer fun, and lots of learning, too, the North American Vegetarian Society Summerfest at the University of Pittsburgh at Johnstown has provided an annual week or weekend (you pick) of sleepaway camp for grown-ups and families for over forty years. Social and educational programming happens there almost around the clock, and Summerfest singles events have made for numerous matches and marriages.

A: Add More to Your Life Than You Subtract

I love this one. It is true that there are lots of common foods that aren't part of a Good Karma Diet. There are also shoes you'll leave in the store because they're made from somebody else's skin, and favorite cosmetics you'll move away from because that company cruelly tests their products on rabbits and others who did not volunteer. But the pleasure of this way of living comes not from what we avoid but from what we embrace. In other words, add more to your life than you subtract.

In the culinary sense alone, most vegans find that the tempting variety of fruits, vegetables, grains, legumes, nuts, seeds, and wonderful specialty and ethnic dishes more than makes up for the foods they no longer eat. You can start to add new foods and habits that promote health and beauty even before you've transitioned away from some of the foods you're looking to leave behind. Many people find that as they add a daily fresh juice, a yummy green smoothie, and the rest of those ten fruits and vegetables we're supposed to consume each day, the subtracting largely takes care of itself.

Discovering the world of vegan fashion—we'll go into detail in chapter 23—is another way to add on. My husband, not the *GQ* type at all, stepped out of character to buy a fedora from Brave Gentle-Man, a designer vegan menswear brand. He paid more than a not-very-metrosexual guy otherwise might, figuring he was supporting the kind of business we want to see flourish, and it's been such fun to see him sporting his hat and enjoying the attention. More than once in a conversation I've heard him say, "We haven't talked about my hat yet."

"Adding" doesn't have to equate with spending money, of course. You can get into gardening, volunteering, or cooking at home more often, and as a result add to both your life and your savings account. This has to be fun. Sure, sometimes there are aggravations—most of my aggravating times, in terms of being vegan, anyway, are at airports and on interstates, places where the food selection can be limited—but there are far more blessings. It's good to stop every now and then and count them.

N: Never Forget the Animals

Someone who eats three times a day and lives to be eighty-five will consume 93,075 meals. That's a lot of breakfasts, lunches, and dinners. A handful will be memorable. A few will be laughingly awful. The vast majority, however, will fade into nothingness in a very short time. But if there was an animal, or a piece of one, on the plate, that was it. That was life. And that was death.

The reason that "Never Forget the Animals" is a vital part of the word "vegan" is because that animal has so much more invested in your meal than you do. For you, it's one of 93,075. For him, or her, and for the mother or the baby left behind, it's one in one. All and everything. If you never forget the animals, you'll always remember why you're doing this.

Camille's Good Karma Story

. . . .

I was already a longtime vegetarian when I signed up to volunteer at Sadhana Forest, a reforestation project and vegan community near Pondicherry in Tamil Nadu, India. Founded by Yorit and Aviram Rozin in 2003, Sadhana Forest draws environmentalists from all over the world, and the Ayurvedic vegan food is just as vibrant and varied as the volunteers who prepare and savor it. Mealtimes are social and sacred at the same time, with a moment of grateful silence before someone sounds a chime and everyone happily tucks in. Sadhana means "spiritual practice" in Sanskrit, and it's a fitting name for a place that will change your life if you let it.

Before my arrival at Sadhana Forest, it hadn't occurred to me that I wasn't actually joking about being addicted to cheese. I'd reached a point at which I felt a vague unease whenever I consumed an omelet or my favorite Cotswold cheddar, and I was excited to be joining a vegan community. I didn't experience an epiphany, however, until a longterm volunteer struck up a conversation at dinnertime. He gently asked what was holding me back from going vegan, and I said I worried about what would happen when family or friends invited me over for dinner—that I might alienate or inconvenience them. "I hear what you're saying," he replied, "but do you see how small a concern that is compared to the abuse animals suffer for our food, and what animal agriculture is doing to the planet?"

In that moment I made the commitment, but I didn't anticipate the magnitude of the change I'd experience over the next few weeks. Up to that point in my career as a novelist, I invariably "suffered" trough periods in between books, periods of frustration that could last up to two years. I was in the middle of one of these troughs at the time of my trip to India, but it had never occurred to me that my diet might have an effect on my creative life.

Sadhana cooks don't use much salt—instead, a salt dish is passed around at lunch and dinner—but I never took any, so I was too low on electrolytes and came down with sunstroke a few days after I decided to go vegan. Tossing and turning under a mosquito net in the "healing hut," I felt depleted and full to bursting at the same time. Whenever I surfaced out of a fever dream, I reached for my journal. The ideas kept coming—ideas for everything, novels and short stories and blog posts and recipes I might invent or reinvent. Best of all, a novel idea I'd been mulling over for a long time finally resolved itself in two simple words: gothic satire. As everyone who makes art knows, that "click" moment can be aggravatingly elusive, but when it does happen, the elation that comes afterward is the best feeling there is. That sickness was a gift.

Has going vegan made me more creative? I've certainly enjoyed unprecedented productivity since my time at Sadhana Forest; I've written three novels in three years (and published my first short story) without so much as a daylong "trough." Fear and uncertainty are no longer an inevitable part of my creative process, perhaps because I am no longer consuming the fear and grief of cows whose babies have been taken from them. The mystery is still there—it always will be!—but today I experience it joyfully.

—**Camille DeAngelis**, VLCE, writer whose latest novel is *Bones & All*. CometParty.com

21

......

Awesome Ancestors

Vegans get excited every time a celebrity takes the plunge. How can we help it? One popular entertainer can influence more people than a hundred committed activists. And we're also cautious. Being pop royalty demands that its sovereigns cycle through changes—fashions, hairstyles, love interests, fitness fads, and dietary samplings—faster than the culture around them. Many contemporary celebrities remain stalwart vegans; others drop by, stay for a while, and move on. We don't have to worry about that with our awesome ancestors, historic vegetarians, some of whom were vegan before the word was coined over seventy years ago.

Going way back, we find Pythagoras, whom I'm crazy about, even though he was into geometry, which I took during summer school so it wouldn't mess up my grade point average. Pythagoras was the first veggie rock star. Yep, the guy with the theorem was, as far as we can tell, vegan (he did eat honey; many modern vegans don't) and a vocal proponent of raw (he called them "unfired") foods. Before students were accepted into his tutelage, they had to agree to a forty-day fast (that's water, not apple/carrot/beet juice) and thereafter adhere to what we would today call a raw vegan diet.

A lot of people don't know that Pythagoras was not only a mathematician and philosopher but also an athletic coach. His most illustrious protégé in sport was Milo of Croton, a wrestler who, on his mentor's unfired vegetable-kingdom diet, won the gold in six Olympiads and chalked up a noteworthy military record besides.

Around the same time, in a different part of the world, the *ahimsa*-based religions—Hinduism, Buddhism, Jainism, and yoga (not a religion but close)—held sway. *Ahimsa* literally means "non-killing" but has long been expanded to mean "harmlessness in thought, word, and deed," and "proactive helpfulness" besides. Rather as Moses brought the Ten Commandments down from Mount Sinai, the *ahimsa* faiths have a series of moral precepts, but this first one outshines the rest.

The late Rynn Berry, undisputed historian of the vegetarian movement, brought this to life for his audiences by explaining that if *ahimsa*-based believers met a hunter in the woods, they could disregard the proscription against lying and tell the hunter that the deer had gone the other way. They could also ignore the injunction against stealing, and filch the hunter's bow when he wasn't looking. If all else failed, they could even disobey the ordinance calling for sexual purity and seduce the hunter, because saving the life of the deer—practicing *ahimsa*—honored the crowning commandment.

Moving ahead in history, the majority of humans around the world likely existed almost entirely on plant foods because, for the poor (and most people were), this was the food available. Outside those areas influenced by Hinduism or Buddhism, however, those who had a choice in the matter and opted for vegetarian fare were few and far between through the late Roman Empire and the Dark and Middle Ages. We don't know for certain that Saint Francis was vegetarian, although it would be an odd carnivore who preached to the birds and purportedly convinced a wolf to cease raiding a village, after extracting from the townspeople a promise to keep the hungry animal fed.

When West Met East

Leonardo da Vinci was almost certainly vegetarian—the explorer Andrea Corsali vouched that he was—but it was the colonizing English, who learned about vegetarianism from the Hindus and Jains they encountered in India, who brought the concept of a meat-free life to the West. Exposure to these ideas was available to anyone who could read English. Those who took to the idea in their libraries and extended it to their kitchens included the poet Shelley and his wife, *Frankenstein* author Mary Shelley, and Leo Tolstoy in Russia, who wrote, ". . . if [a man] eats meat, he participates in taking animal life merely for the sake of his appetite. And to act so is immoral."

British writers and educators spread their influence to America, as well. The Bible Christian Church included vegetarianism among its tenets and was popular in both the United Kingdom and the United States in the 1800s. It had been brought to America by Reverend William Metcalfe, who joined with Presbyterian minister Sylvester Graham and others to found the first American Vegetarian Society in 1850. Graham was instrumental in the "health reform" movement of that era, invented Graham bread (whole-grain, in response to the new trend toward white-flour products), and was such a threat to established industries that in 1837 a coalition of Boston butchers and bakers formed to prevent him from speaking there.

Ellen G. White, one of the founders of the Seventh Day Adventist Church in 1863, had revelations that told her that the ideal diet for humans was the original one given to Adam and Eve in Genesis 1:29: "Then God said, 'Behold, I give you every plant yielding seed that is on the surface of all the earth, and every tree which has fruit yielding seed; it shall be food for you.'"

White wrote about a vegetarian and even "pure" vegetarian (no animal products) diet, and about eating foods in their intact state. Although adopting vegetarianism has never been required for church membership, about 50 percent of Adventists are practicing vegetarians, and about half of those are vegans. Loma Linda, California, site of Adventist institutions Loma Linda University and Loma Linda School of Medicine, is North America's only "Blue Zone," a place where the average inhabitant lives longer and in better health than his or her counterpart elsewhere.

Dipping back into history again, Adventist John Harvey Kellogg (1852–1943) was a GI surgeon who championed breathing exercises, temperance, and a whole-food, vegetarian diet, crediting its high-fiber and lower-protein content with preventing the digestive disorders that had resulted in his bustling surgery practice. Celebrities who flocked to his Battle Creek, Michigan, sanitarium included vegetarians George Bernard Shaw and *Tarzan* actor Johnny Weissmuller, as well as Amelia Earhart, Thomas Edison, and Henry Ford, who "took the cure" but stopped short of a plant-based conversion.

GKT

Umami, an enticing flavor imparted by the amino acid glutamate, may be the "something missing" that certain people long for when they go vegan. Virginia Messina, MPH, RD, recommends satisfying an umami craving with fermented foods (wine, tamari, miso, sauerkraut), fresh tomatoes and ketchup, dried sea vegetables, mushrooms, olives, nutritional yeast, and balsamic vinegar. Vegan cheeses also hit the umami spot.

In the twentieth century, and from the Indian subcontinent itself, came Mahatma Gandhi. He had given up his Hindu family's traditional vegetarian diet as a young attorney living abroad but returned to it as he came to realize that violence is violence, whether inflicted upon a human or an animal. In his later life, he wanted desperately to be vegan, but youthful overindulgence in the fiery spices of his homeland had left him with a stomach that could handle only the blandest of foods, and in those days before plant milks, his doctors insisted that he consume goat's milk. The Mahatma, "great soul," called this "the tragedy of my life."

Gandhi's writings on nonviolence and civil disobedience influenced Martin Luther King Jr., and Dr. King, in turn, influenced Dick Gregory, a hugely popular (and morbidly obese) comedian in the 1960s. Gregory became deeply involved in the American civil rights movement and was inspired to read Gandhi for himself. He went vegetarian and ultimately adopted a raw, vegan diet with lots of juicing.

He lost the weight and spread the vegan message in comedy shows, campus lectures, and his 1974 book, *Dick Gregory's Natural Diet for Folks Who Eat*. Ever the funny man, Gregory hid a joke in his title. Known for fasting and juice fasting, he stipulated that the book was for "folks who eat," alluding to the fact that he himself often didn't. Now in his eighties, Mr. Gregory still travels extensively to speak and perform.

Veganism Gets Its Name

While some earlier vegetarians had eschewed eggs and dairy, as well, it was in the mid-1940s that the concept of veganism was solidified by Donald Watson and his wife, Dorothy, who together coined the term. They were part of a group of English vegetarians who had come to see that avoiding veal, the by-product of dairying, while consuming the milk that caused the veal industry to exist, was ethically and pragmatically inconsistent. This small band of caring people started The Vegan Society (VeganSociety.com) in 1944.

The late H. Jay Dinshah and his bride, Freya, launched the American Vegan Society (AmericanVegan.org) in 1960 in Malaga, New Jersey, near Philadelphia. It was their writings, and their patience with me as a young and recalcitrant would-be vegan, that are behind the life I have today and the book you're reading now. AVS is going strong under the leadership of Mrs. Dinshah and her daughter, Anne.

GKT

Given the abundance of plant-powered cookbooks on the market, it's hard to believe that not so long ago, there were only a handful. The ones that taught me to cook and eat as a vegan were *The Vegan Kitchen*, by Freya Dinshah; *Ten Talents*, by Rosalie and Dr. Frank Hurd; *The Peaceful Palate*, by Jennifer Raymond; *The American Vegetarian Cookbook from the Fit for Life Kitchen*, by Marilyn Diamond; and *The Compassionate Cook*, by Ingrid Newkirk. I still use all of these today.

In 1971, The Farm, a vegan commune in Tennessee, was established by hippie prophet Stephen Gaskin. Although much smaller now than in its heyday, it has survived and spreads its influence through the Book Publishing Company, a highly vegan-centric publishing house responsible for such genre best-sellers as Ellen Jaffe Jones's *Eat Vegan on $4 a Day* and Jennifer Cornbleet's *Raw Food Made Easy for 1 or 2 People*.

On the raw food front, the American Natural Hygiene Society was formed back in 1948 with Dr. Herbert Shelton, author of *Fasting Can Save Your Life*, and other alternative health pioneers at its helm.

The philosophy was clean living, a diet high in raw, plant foods, and supervised fasting to allow the body to heal itself. (ANHS went through a reconfiguration process and is now the National Health Association, HealthScience.org.) In 1962, Lithuanian immigrant Ann Wigmore, affectionately known to thousands of followers as Dr. Ann, started the original Hippocrates Health Institute in Boston. She introduced the world to wheatgrass juice and popularized sprouting. Her legacy continues at the Ann Wigmore Institute in Puerto Rico (AnnWigmore.org) and the Hippocrates Health Institute in West Palm Beach, Florida (HippocratesInst.org).

The Power of the Pen

Books have always propelled this movement forward, and a host of American titles in the late twentieth century laid the groundwork for the surge of plant-based eating and cruelty-free living we see today. Although some of my contemporaries might compile a different list, these are the titles I see as pivotal:

- *Eating for Life*, by Nathaniel Altman, debuted in 1973 as the first non-self-published work on vegetarianism to appear in America since the 1800s. The author and I worked at the same spiritual center in Illinois: he typed his first drafts on a manual typewriter, and I copied the chapters on the fancy IBM electric typewriter in my office.

- *Dick Gregory's Natural Diet for Folks Who Eat* (1974) introduced raw foods, juicing, and animal-free eating to the African American community and the country at large.

- *Diet for a Small Planet*, by Frances Moore Lappé. This 1975 bestseller tied modern livestock production to world hunger and put vegetarian eating on the map.

- *Animal Liberation*, by Peter Singer. This Australian philosopher's seminal work taught the world a new term and presented a new concept: "animal rights." The book came out in 1975, one year after the North American Vegetarian Society was founded and *Vegetarian Times* magazine began publication. PETA would come on the scene in 1980.

- *Fit for Life*, by Harvey and Marilyn Diamond. This 1985 blockbuster espousing a high-raw and nearly vegan diet accounted for a 10 percent uptick in U.S. fruit and vegetable sales for two years running. Its worldwide sales are in the multimillions.

- *Compassion the Ultimate Ethic: An Exploration of Veganism*, my undergraduate thesis, was published in book form by Thorsons (UK), Ltd., in 1985. Its worldwide sales were paltry, but it has historic value as the first book on vegan philosophy and practice to come from an actual publishing house. When it went out of print, the American Vegan Society took it over and sells it to this day.

- *Diet for a New America*, by John Robbins, brought everything full circle in 1987 with a powerful read connecting the way we treat animals, the way we treat our bodies, and the fate of the planet. The author, who had walked away from an ice cream fortune to become a visionary, increased the vegan ranks significantly so that when the twenty-first century brought an explosion of vegan books, cookbooks, food products, clothing lines, cosmetics, and household products, there was a customer base—and a mentor base for the masses of new vegans showing up.

- *Dr. Dean Ornish's Program for Reversing Heart Disease* became a *New York Times* bestseller in 1990. It details the diet (vegetarian, low-fat, minimal amounts of low-fat dairy and egg whites) and lifestyle intervention (yoga, meditation, gentle exercise, and group support) Dr. Ornish used to show for the first time that coronary heart disease could be reversed. A devoted yoga practitioner as well as an innovative medical doctor and researcher, Ornish had wanted to call the book *Opening Your Heart*, a true statement on many levels.

- *Mad Cowboy*, by Howard Lyman, hit the shelves in 1998, telling the story of the Montana rancher-turned-vegan who was sued along with Oprah Winfrey in the 1996 meat defamation lawsuit filed by the Texas Beef Group. It took years of litigation, but Big Beef lost and free speech won.

All these authors are still alive, so they're only ideologically ancestral, but this overview gives a cursory look at a few of the people who discovered and championed a plant-based diet and cruelty-free lifestyle when both were relatively unknown. The list of vegetarians is much longer and includes men and women representing a multitude of times, places, and pursuits. We have Diogenes and Marcus Aurelius, Charlotte Brontë and Harriet Beecher Stowe. In the twentieth century, we added Cesar Chavez and Rosa Parks, and Drs. Albert Schweitzer and Benjamin Spock. And if you look up "famous vegetarians" or "famous vegans," you'll see impressive lists of present-day luminaries in sports and the arts, science and medicine, business and technology. Their reach is extensive and their influence is strong, and so is yours.

We can fail to recognize in the midst of our lives how many others we touch and how many people observe our actions and note our progress. It will not go unnoticed when you get healthier and happier and start to shine with an inner light that's brighter than it's ever been. That's enough to pique the interest of someone in your world who is looking for a bigger life or a better one. And the first time you ignite a spark in a burger-and-fries guy you never expected to come in this direction, it could feel downright historic.

22

······

Plant-Built Muscle

I was easy to spot in school: the chubby kid who always volunteered to stay in from recess and help the teacher staple quizzes or wash the chalkboards. That saved me from the humiliation of being chosen last for whatever impromptu team was forming, or from the outright assault of dodgeball. To a kid like that, "Let's go out and play" never sounds appealing. Even today, when the preternaturally good-natured twentysomething behind the desk at the gym says, "Have a good workout," my first thought tends to be: "Seriously? Jane Austen is 'good.' So is a movie with more dialogue than special effects, and delicious conservation at a quiet restaurant. Being bored out of my mind for an hour on a stationary bike doesn't come close."

But you know what? When I'm working out consistently and get into the groove of the thing, I do have a good workout. When it's over, and I realize that even though conventional wisdom says I'll never build much muscle—I'm female, and vegan, and sixty-four like the Beatles song—I have indeed built muscle. And my aspirations here in late middle age include no plans, in the words of Paul McCartney, "to rent a cottage on the Isle of Wight." There's too much to do that's exciting—and important.

The idea that you have to eat animal muscle to build your muscle is a myth, like the old tribal belief that eating the heart of a slain enemy imparts his courage to the surviving warrior. Both notions make sense on some level, but then, the earth looks flat, too. The fact of this matter was perhaps stated best by Pam Popper, ND (she's coauthor of *Food over Medicine*), when she said, "You don't build muscle in the kitchen. You build muscle in the gym." Of course you need something from which to build it, and that means you have to eat enough food. When you get enough calories from whole plant foods to fuel the life you've chosen, you'll also get enough of the constituent nutrients—protein included—to fuel that life.

GKT

Do whatever it takes to get you moving. Have a buddy you'll meet at the track. Work overtime to pay for a trainer. If you have to, sleep in your workout clothes so you won't have an excuse in the morning (just don't tell anyone it was me who told you to do that).

Where Fitness Fits In

Do you have to work out to eat a Good Karma Diet? No. But if you want all the good karma that's yours to collect, it's indispensable. You see, your body has needs the way your car has needs. You can put in the right gasoline, rotate the tires, and detail that baby so it looks brand-new, but if you never get an oil change, you're going to have car trouble.

Your body is counting on you to provide it with high-quality food; sufficient rest and sleep; protection from toxins; a positive mental attitude that seeps into your very cells; love and meaning and community; and regular, sometimes rigorous, physical activity. If you're lacking one or two of these, having the others helps take up the slack. For example, if you eat well and you have a lot of inner peace, one night with less sleep than you need won't matter much. If, however, you're poorly nourished and a bundle of nerves, missing out on a single night's shut-eye could put enough stress on your system that you come down with whatever virus is making the rounds.

Food is important and so is exercise. The latter gets more valuable as we age, when letting nature take its course would mean less muscle, less bone mass, less energy, and less ability to catch ourselves and intercept a fall. Does failing to exercise lead to *more* of anything? Oh yeah: more fat and more likelihood of succumbing to type 2 diabetes, Alzheimer's, some cancers, and the inglorious catchall, "premature death."

Move Your Body, Change Your Life

So, what kind of exercise would I recommend? Well, the kind you like, if there is one, or the kind you'll tolerate, if there isn't. Who are you? Do you have a strong competitive side? Are you attracted to something expressive like dance or some discipline, such as a martial art? Are you goal-oriented, so that even thinking you might one day do a Tough Mudder race will get you to the gym? Or are you simply pragmatic and willing to do perfunctory cardio, strength training, and stretching regularly for the sake of your health?

I'm in that last category. And because I'm far more intrigued by the mysteries of life (Why are we here? What's it all about? Show me the Big Picture!) than about my aerobic training zone, I've found it helpful to see the metaphysical and metaphorical underpinnings of cardio, resistance training, and stretching.

The continuous movement of walking, running, dancing, cycling, and swimming that counts for cardio is also sometimes called "endurance exercise," and I like to think, when I've been on the treadmill for twenty-seven minutes and forty-five seems as if it will never come, that I'm not just strengthening my cardiorespiratory system but building endurance for life overall. I focus, when I'd rather be doing anything besides putting one foot in front of the other, on staying the course, keeping the commitment, and coming through for myself, whether on this artificial hike or my actual trek through life.

Strength training has a metaphysical and metaphorical underside, as well: the way it builds unseen strength to face what's frightening. At one point when I was working out a lot and taking self-defense classes, I noticed, as I drove down a street in Kansas City, a man punching a woman, right there on the sidewalk. There were plenty of pedestrians, but they just watched. I got out of my car, walked right up to the guy (who, I realized as I got close, was enormous), and screamed at the top of my lungs: "Cut it out!"

Those three loud words rendered Goliath speechless. He moved his mouth, but no words came. At twice his age and half his size, I'd scared the stuffing out of the guy. The unfortunate postscript is that the woman got up on her tiptoes—did I say this lout was big?—and kissed him on the cheek. Shoot. But she'd seen me confront him and I want to believe that planted a seed within her that she deserved better. I'm not implying that just because you can do a few push-ups means you're supposed to become a vigilante, only that when you feel strong, you can deal with the scary stuff, whether in the form of a big-sized bully or a business-sized envelope.

Stretching, yoga, ballet—the kind of movement that keeps you pliant and pliable, preventing injury and putting off the aches and pains we're supposed to expect at a certain point—become metaphysical and metaphorical when you see that flexibility is also about becoming internally resilient.

I was once at a low-cost Scandinavian furniture store, returning a desk I'd bought. It seemed to have come in eight thousand pieces, and I was supposed to put it together with a strange little tool shaped like an "L." No way. To return the thing, I'd had to make a second trek to New Jersey, rehiring the guy who'd driven me out there the first time, "Schmuck with a Truck." The take-back line looked as if it reached Saturn. I was angry and tense and could feel my shoulders hunching, my jaws clenching, and my forehead wrinkling in that way that explains the popularity of Botox.

It must have been the appropriate response in the take-back line, though, because everybody there was hunched and clenched and wrinkled—everybody, that is, except for one woman of thirty or maybe thirty-five. She appeared perfectly relaxed as she did side bends and pliés and relevés, as if she was in ballet class in Paris or Moscow, not in the return line at a Big Box store in the suburbs.

That was when it hit me like a ton of pointe shoes: when the body is flexible, the mind is more likely to be flexible. Wherever you are, in whatever situation, you can tense up and resist, or loosen up and flow. Everybody in that queue eventually made it to the counter, but the ballet lady, unlike the rest of us, did so with poise and peace. That's why yoga is big on stretching: the goal of yoga is poise and peace; a brain that lives in a relaxed and limber body is likely to have those as its default.

GKT

Working out is half the equation; recovery is the other. Elite athletes have known this for years, and the rest of us can join them by following a hard workout with a magnesium-rich Epsom salts bath, a sauna and/or massage, lots of hydration, or a protein-rich smoothie within twenty minutes of a run or lifting session.

100% Performance, 0% Cruelty

That's the tag line on shirts from Athletica-V, a vegan-owned and vegan-principled athletic clothing company. It's also the doctrine behind plant-fueled athletes tearing up the record books in nearly every sport. While their numbers are markedly increasing, vegan athletes are not a new phenomenon. Carl Lewis made Olympic history on a plant-based diet; Georges Laraque is a hockey legend; and Martina Navratilova extended her championship career under the tutelage of raw vegan mentor Dr. Douglas Graham. (His book, *Nutrition and Athletic Performance*, is a game changer, whether you're a professional athlete or you just like Zumba.)

Former pro Ironman Brendan Brazier is now an author (of *Thrive: The Vegan Nutrition Guide to Optimal Performance in Sports and Life*, and *Thrive Energy Cookbook*), lecturer, and businessman (he is the owner of Vega, an all-vegan line of athletic supplement powders and snacks). After John Salley left the NBA, he began vegan pursuits in earnest. The competitive career of bodybuilder Jim Morris spanned five decades and, at seventy-eight, he now trains others.

To follow is a highly abridged scorecard of some of our plant-powered superstars and their fields of endeavor. (Thanks to Robert Cheeke, author of *Vegan Bodybuilding and Fitness* and *Shred It!*, and a runner and champion bodybuilder himself, for help putting together this list.)

Austin Aries, pro wrestler
Patrik Baboumian, strongman
Ed Bauer, bodybuilder
Rob Bigwood, arm wrestler
David Carter, NFL defensive tackle
Matt Danzig, MMA fighter
Glen Davis, NBA star

Meagan Duhamel, Olympic figure skating silver medalist
MaryJo Cooke Elliott, IFBB pro figure competitor
Matt Frazier, ultramarathoner
Ruth Heidrich, masters level endurance running champion
Keith Holmes, boxer
Ellen Jaffe Jones, masters level champion sprinter
James Jones, two-time NBA champion
Scott Jurek, ultramarathon champion
Laura Kline, World Champion duathlete
Jeremy Moore, national level cyclist and speed skater
Fiona Oakes, World Champion ultra-runner
Montell Owens, NFL running back
Rich Roll, elite endurance runner
Ronda Rousey, judo champion and extreme fighter
Jake Shields, MMA fighter
Bill Simmonds, Mr. Universe
Amar'e Stoudemire, NBA star
Ed Templeton, skateboarder
Hannah Teter, snowboarder
Will Tucker, champion professional bodybuilder
Alexey Voyevoda, three-time world champion arm wrestler
    and Olympic Gold medal–winning bobsledder
Torre Washington, champion professional bodybuilder
Serena Williams, tennis champion
Venus Williams, tennis champion

Each one of these people has a compelling story and a unique character that pushes them to endure grueling workouts and to opt for a compassionate diet, sometimes against the vigorous opposition of trainers and teammates. One of my favorite stories is that of the English marathoner Fiona Oakes. During a single year, she ran full marathons on all seven continents plus the North Pole—she was the fastest woman there—*and she doesn't even like to run*. She does it to draw attention to the efficacy of a vegan diet, and to help support her sanctuary for rescued horses and farmed animals, Tower Hill Stables, in the Essex countryside. And, oh, yes: as the result of a childhood accident, she has an artificial knee.

You may also want to become acquainted with the PlantBuilt Team, an official coterie of imposing vegan bodybuilders, physique and figure athletes, CrossFit-ers, and powerlifters, male and female, who defy the stereotype that you can't build muscle on "incomplete" plant protein. They're currently competing, and they check in, along with us mere mortals, as part of Robert Cheeke's Vegan Bodybuilding & Fitness Facebook group, providing great inspiration on those days when writing off exercise seems like a perfectly reasonable thing to do.

Some days, it actually *is* wise to skip your workout, such as when you're newly injured or know you're coming down with something; and there is such a thing as "exercise bulimia," working out to extremes or beyond what's required to prepare for a competition. There are far fewer exercise bulimics, however, than there are people who suffer from "activity resistance disorder." I came up with that term myself, but even if the phrase isn't for real, the state of mind is. I've had it plenty of times: "I hurt my shoulder; I can't walk on a treadmill . . . It's raining; I have to watch TV . . . I skipped the gym yesterday; I may as well sit out today."

People with an athletic mind-set train the way I eat. Although I long since let go of binge eating, I eat every day. I may be short on time or short on money, under the weather or over the moon, but I'll find a way to get some food. The admirably fit may do that, too, but they're equally determined to work out, and they're helping me build that same determination. I think all of us want this deep inside. That's why we admire athletes so much, and why Nike's "Just Do It" slogan became almost instantly iconic: exerciser or non-exerciser, everybody knew that this was all there was to it.

For those prone to activity resistance disorder (I'll bet if we started calling it ARD, it would really catch on), *Vegan Health and Fitness Magazine* is a great inspiration. And for those who already get it that sweating for the better part of an hour almost every day is the rent we're expected to pay for being housed in these bodies, the magazine is a terrific resource on all things fit and sporting in the plant-based world.

Whatever gets you moving is valid, whether it's competitiveness, vanity, or even fear. "Every adult woman in my family of origin had cancer," says champion sprinter and recreational distance runner Ellen Jaffe Jones. "I'm running for my life out there." In the Good Karma sense, however, the real point of all the sweating and lifting and stretching is this: When you have what others want—in this case, an enviable degree of fitness—they'll do what you did to get it. And what you'll do as a vegan is mitigate suffering and give future generations a fighting chance. If you can bring folks around because you finish a race or you have great-looking arms, that's a victory.

Mike's Good Karma Story

In 2008, I ate about 2,500 pounds of meat. I was also a hard-core drug and alcohol addict, and spent more than $1,000 a week getting those fixes. Looking back on my life and what I had become—a 550-pound monster that only cared about my gluttony and addiction—I attempted suicide by swallowing a concoction of forty Vicodin pills and a bottle of whiskey, hoping that I would die in my sleep and feel no more pain.

I woke up three days later, in a desperate state and needing medical attention, but I was so out of my mind and had such complete loss of motor functioning that I couldn't even dial 911 for help. I needed a miracle to happen, just to feel human again.

In the first week of January 2009, I decided to check myself into rehab. Before going, however, *The Wrestler*, a feature film starring Mickey Rourke, came out in the theaters and many of my friends were excited because they had seen my little part in the movie as a "wrestler in the crowd." That sparked something in my brain, and I thought that rehab was not the best route for me to heal, so instead I found a wrestling school and started training to be a professional wrestler. Seriously—this is the way I beat my addiction.

But one month into my training, my body—still in the process of detoxifying heavily—was having a difficult time recovering from the intense training required to be a professional athlete. Starting to sink into depression again, I began to contemplate another way to end my life. Then, out of nowhere, I met a woman who would change my life forever. She had been a vegetarian for fifteen years, and after hearing about my consumption of 500 to 600 grams of protein a day, she suggested that I cut the meat out of my diet. I chuckled and asked her how the heck I was supposed to get enough protein as a 500-pound wrestler without eating meat. She was quick to send me examples of powerful vegan athletes, including the vegan bodybuilder Robert Cheeke— but I still wasn't convinced I would be strong eating plants.

Then, she decided to send me a video of cute, fuzzy baby chickens being thrown into a meat grinder alive because they were male and couldn't lay eggs. Whatever synapses in my brain had not been firing prior to seeing that video suddenly started working. I watched these beautiful little creatures become pulverized into something that nature never intended. My eyes had opened my heart to the reality that for the first twenty-nine years of my life I had been a taker— not just a taker of animals' lives, but also from the environment. That is when my journey truly began.

For the last several years, I have lived my life with a purpose. I no longer suffer from depression, and my health has been completely restored. Many people have noticed this change, and as a result, I have been interviewed in four documentaries relating to veganism. I am currently in the final stages of my first book, illustrating the journey that I just shared with you. I am vegan for the animals, the environment, and my health.

—**Big Bald Mike**, The World's Unlikeliest Vegan.
www.bigbaldmike.com

23
......

Beauty, Fashion, and Good Karma Shopping

t's not just food. All our actions, all our purchases, and all our intentions can contribute to creating a more heavenly earth: kind, clean, peaceful, safe. I used to shop for recreation: "This looks cute," or "I want one of those," or "That's on sale." Over time, the act of shopping has become a more conscious, even meaningful, part of the magnificent mandate to lessen the suffering that permeates our world. And you know what? Just as food tastes better than it ever did, shopping is even more fun than it was in the old days.

When it's time to send a gift and I opt for extraordinary sweets from Allison's Gourmet (AllisonsGourmet.com) or luxurious natural toiletries from Fanciful Fox (FancifulFox.bigcartel.com); or I surprise a good friend's best friend with vegan doggy treats from Boston Baked Bonz (BostonBakedBonz.com), I'm gifting them with something wonderful, while also gifting myself with the good feeling of sharing this lifestyle in a way that's not even borderline pushy. I'm also supporting a company that's committed to making life better for all beings.

When shopping brick-and-mortar, I pay attention and read labels, not only to see if an item is technically vegan (no animal products, no animal testing) but also whether it's safe for the planet and for me, and where it was made. A sweatshop garment may be cheap enough that I could buy two, but that's not how I want to spend my money. The result is that I have fewer clothes and fewer objects overall, but more clothes and more objects that give me real pleasure.

Conscious shopping is something anyone can begin right now, even if they're not ready for major changes in their diet. I went to dinner a while back with a lovely friend of mine, Barbara Biziou— you might know her work as an author and spiritual teacher (BarbaraBiziou.com). Anyway, she'd invited her former college roommate to join us and when it came out that I'm a vegan, the room-mate said, "I'm a vegan, too." Barbara looked surprised. "You are? I didn't know that." And her friend replied, "Well, I don't *eat* vegan, but all my cosmetics and toiletries are vegan." Come to find out, she's a distributor for Arbonne, a company that manufactures top-of-the-line, cruelty-free, natural cosmetics. Who'd have thought that, at least in some settings, being vegan would be sufficiently cool to prompt an expansion of the definition?

GKT

Have fun with kitchen cosmetics. Black tea bags dampened with cold water can relieve puffy eyes. Oats, ground to a fine powder in your blender, are a skin-soothing addition to your bath. Coconut oil is an all-purpose makeup remover and moisturizer, and canned coconut milk is a terrific hair conditioner.

But, you know, she was right in a way: just as some health vegans eat plant foods but otherwise live conventionally, she got her foot in the door as a makeup-and-skin-care vegan. This means the door is open now, a very good thing. There are three reasons for being a makeup vegan (and a toothpaste/shaving cream/deodorant vegan):

1. Most cosmetic products, especially those from huge corporations, the ones you find most readily in drugstore chains and discount houses, department stores and cosmetic emporia, are tested on animals in ways only a sadistic psychopath would enjoy hearing described.

2. Toiletries may contain animal ingredients including, but not limited to, cow's or goat's milk derivatives, carmine (a red coloring made from ground-up insects), lanolin (from sheep's wool), bee products including honey, beeswax, or royal jelly, and occasionally fish oils or fish eggs.

3. Many conventional cosmetics contain questionable chemicals that enter the body through your skin. (See the Environmental Working Group's "Skin Deep" program, which tracks the toxicity level of nearly seventy thousand products: ewg.org.) Companies that identify as vegan are likely to avoid harmful chemicals, as well; and those companies that may not be fully vegan but are conscientious enough to do safety testing without the use of live animals are also more likely than their competitors to keep potentially harmful ingredients out of their products. As a general rule, cosmetic and body care items sold in a natural food store stand a good chance of being both cruelty-free and nontoxic.

Red fruits and vegetables—pomegranate, tomatoes, beets, etc.—contain lycopene, an antioxidant that increases collagen production for younger-looking skin. Other collagen boosters are soy foods, leafy greens, and legumes.

Animal testing, with all its attendant horror, is not required by law in the United States or Canada, and it's actually banned by the EU. Humane methods are more modern and far more dependable, but some companies persist in the old ways because it's what they've always done. Others who had ceased animal testing at one point went back to the practice in order to get their products into China, where laws required it. PETA and some other groups are working to develop non-animal tests that will satisfy the Chinese government. Progress has been made on that front and, even more exciting, animal rights proponents working toward these ends report that many people in the cosmetics and household products industries also want animal testing to become a thing of the past.

Until it does, the specifics—which companies test on animals, which don't—change with some frequency. The LeapingBunny.org site, curated by a coalition of animal rights organizations, can be invaluable for staying abreast of which companies have beautiful policies as well as glamorous products. The Leaping Bunny app is available for the iPhone and Android, so you can confirm a company's status while you shop. And a terrific vegan beauty blog for keeping up with it all is LogicalHarmony.com.

While many companies do not engage in animal testing, some almost hide the fact. When possible, I prefer to support the ones that make a big whoop-de-do about it on their websites. I want to see the Leaping Bunny logo, a recognized symbol for companies that avoid animal testing, on the label; or the proud statement "No animal testing," "Cruelty-free," or, best of all, "Vegan," which means no testing *and* no animal ingredients. It's companies like these that you can count on to *stay* cruelty-free. Most of them also require that their suppliers not engage in animal testing.

To follow is a short list—there are many more, and others coming all the time—of full-line cosmetics companies (those with at least some makeup as well as face/body and/or hair care products) that let the world know that cruelty-free is the way to be. *Not all the companies listed are entirely vegan.* I've included them because they're vocal about their non-testing stance and/or because their products are widely available.

- Arbonne
- Ava Anderson
- Beauty Without Cruelty
- The Body Shop
- Colorganics (including Hemp Organics)
- Dr. Hauschka
- Ecco Bella
- E.L.F. (eyes, lips, face)
- Gabriel Cosmetics, Inc. (including Zuzu Luxe)
- GlamNatural
- Jane Iredale
- LUSH
- Modern Minerals
- Mün
- MyChelle Dermaceuticals
- Neal's Yard Remedies
- Nvey Eco
- Obsessive Compulsive Cosmetics
- Paul Penders
- Urban Decay

Among the clean, cruelty-free companies that manufacture skin care, hair care, and/or body care products, but not makeup, are:

- Ahava Dead Sea Laboratories
- Alba Botanica
- Aubrey
- Avalon Organics
- Burt's Bees (body care plus lip glosses)
- Christie Brinkley Authentic Skincare
- EO
- Fanciful Fox
- Jāsön
- Nourish Organic
- Ology
- Pangea Organics
- ShiKai
- Yes To (Blueberries, Carrots, Cucumbers, etc.)

And there are specialty companies. LVX, Karma Organic Spa, and Priti NYC specialize in nail lacquers. Hurraw! makes lip balm, and Schmidt's is a natural deodorant. Paul Mitchell specializes in hair care, and their John Paul Pet line offers grooming products for dogs, cats, and horses. PureOlogy Serious Colour Care is another lovely vegan hair care line. Kelley Quan is known for makeup brushes. Harvey Prince formulates luscious fragrances—I love "Ageless," their scent based on research into an "olfactory antidote to aging"; Tom's of Maine is well known for oral care, soap, and deodorant; and there is, of course, the counterculture classic, Dr. Bronner's Magic Soaps.

More companies like these are cropping up. One way to sample a variety of lovely cosmetics is to join Petit Vour (PetitVour.com) and receive a box of luxurious, vegan products—full sizes for nail lacquers, lipstick, serum concentrates, and the like; travel sizes for shampoos, moisturizers, etc.—each month.

Getting beyond cosmetics, you'll want to choose the cleanest cleaning and laundry products, too—those that aren't outgassing fetid fumes and that weren't used to torture the innocent. Readily available brands include BonAmi, Ecover, Method, Mrs. Meyers Clean Day, Ology, and Seventh Generation. And you can clean anything short of a toxic waste dump with white vinegar, dishwashing liquid, club soda, and baking soda (I get Bob's Red Mill—they don't do animal testing—at the health food store). It's actually fun to simplify, and you save money, too.

Vegans in Vogue

Just as eating should be a pleasure, it seems to me that dressing should be fun, and I'm not ashamed to admit to a lifelong love affair with fashion. I figured out early which fashion types I did not relate to. Preppy, even when it matured into classic/corporate with pencil skirts and no-nonsense jackets, headed the "no" list; but ruffled-romantic, and the billowy, peasant-dress, made-in-a-collective-in-Guatemala look, were on it, too. I finally decided to call my style "Euro-indie." If a garment reminds me of Paris in the '20s, London in the '60s, or a designer at a sewing machine in the back of an East Village shop right this minute, I'll probably like it.

Whatever your style, you can flaunt it famously as part of your Good Karma Life. There are even magazines especially for fashion-and-culture-conscious vegans. *Laika* (LaikaMagazine.com) is lovely—think vegan *Vanity Fair*. And for pure fashion and beauty, there are online publications hailing from both sides of the Atlantic. London-based *Vilda* (VildaMagazin.com) and New York's *La Fashionista Compassionista* (LaFCnyc.com) are both glorious; either could become the vegan *Vogue*.

And while not everyone follows fashion, everyone is influenced by it. Menswear designer and fashion academician Joshua Katcher (his blog is TheDiscerningBrute.com) does a riveting presentation for the Main Street Vegan Academy program in which he details how humans have used clothing for millennia to tell others who they are, to express power or lack of it, and to exclude outsiders. Animals have been an unwitting part of this from the beginning. We've used their fur, their skins, their feathers, their wool, and even their babies (Persian lamb, for instance, comes from a newborn or fetal Karakul sheep).

Sometimes living animals are tormented—down or feathers are painfully plucked from live geese, and wool is cruelly shorn from sheep. I know what you're thinking, and I once thought it, too: sheep have to be shorn or they'd get too hot. This is true, but only because we've bred them to be wool machines. And commercial sheepshearing bears scant resemblance to what happens when you take your dog to the groomer. Shearing is about speed, output, and money; casualties of the process are terrified, bleeding, and often injured animals. In Australia, where most wool is produced, lambs are subjected to the heinous practice of mulesing, slicing off the skin of their backsides with no anesthesia, so the hairless, scarred wound will not attract the maggot infestation called fly strike. And sheep raised for wool are eventually slaughtered to be eaten.

Some animals are killed expressly for clothing, e.g., furbearers such as mink and chinchilla, and reptiles such as alligators and snakes, whose skins are prized for "exotic" shoes, purses, and watchbands. Other animals are slaughtered for meat, but because they have parts that can also be used for clothing—leather, calfskin, pigskin, or goose feathers when they are the by-product of the cruel foie gras trade—they keep the cost of meat down and bring more money into the animal-killing business. Once upon a time, it probably was "us or them" and humans needed the skins of animals to survive as they moved northward. Today, we can stay warm and set trends without one iota of animal skin, fur, hair, down, feathers, or silk (the little larvae we call silkworms are boiled to death after doing their job).

If you just can't wait to start shopping, here's a list of online stores that cater to vegans of every taste, from casual to couture:

- AlternativeOutfitters.com
- CompassionCoutureShop
- Foranima.com
- GrapeCat.com
- HerbivoreClothing.com
- MooShoes.com
- VeganEssentials.com
- VeganStore.com
- TheVegetarianSite.com
- YoureSoVegan.co.uk

Shoe Business

Vegans are way past plastic pumps, canvas tennies, and macramé handbags. I think one reason we're sometimes still conflated with hippie culture is that the clothing once available to us made us look hippie-like years after a generation headed to San Francisco with flowers in their hair. These days, however, there are fashionable vegans in San Francisco and everyplace else where people value aesthetics *and* ethics.

It starts from the ground up—well, the feet up. While budget-friendly vegan shoes can be found at PayLess and Target, it's a growing group of committed designers whose shoes and boots create the trends to be copied.. Women's shoes from companies such as Beyond Skin, Cri de Coeur, Elizabeth's Kind Café, Mink Shoes, Neuaura, Nicora Johns, and Olsenhaus make *Sex and the City*'s stilettos so last century. Lines for men include Brave GentleMan (which also has clothing), Freerangers, and NoHarm. Bourgeois Boheme, Novacas,

Opificio V, Vegetarian Shoes, and Wills Animal and Human Friendly Shoes are cobblers to both genders.

In addition to the online vegan shops listed previously, and some freestanding vegan stores, there are also special leather-free sections on the big online shoe sites such as Zappo's.

When I go into a physical shoe store, other than the all-vegan MooShoes on Manhattan's Lower East Side, I smell the shoes to see what's what. Leather reeks, the lingering effect of the toxic process of tanning. In India, the world's number one leather exporter, young boys are often the ones to do this life-shortening work.

Arm Candy

Vegan bags have unmistakably come into their own in recent years. The new fibers—cloth blends, never-before-seen fabrics made from recycled materials, and non-PVC faux leathers—are glorious. When I'm carrying my Jill Milan bag (JillMilan.com) and get a compliment (which always happens), I respond with, "And feel it." I'm probably developing a reputation as that odd woman who wants everybody to touch her pocketbook, but it's worth that risk to share with someone the ultra-soft, rich feel of a bag that is expertly crafted and intentionally vegan.

Wonderful vegan totes, clutches, shoulder bags, cross-body bags, evening bags, man-bags, briefcases, and wallets in a variety of price ranges also come from designers including CoraLlei (CoraLlei .com), Cornelia Guest (CorneliaGuest.com), Matt & Nat (MattandNat .com), Melie Bianco (MelieBianco.com), and Susan Nichole (Susan Nichole.com).

When I was fresh out of high school and headed for fashion college in London (I thought I'd be a fashion coordinator, although to this day I'm not entirely sure what that means), I read an authoritative how-to-dress book. In it the author bluntly, if not personally, informed me: "You're as good as your leather." If I met her today, I'd tell her—wait, I wouldn't tell her anything; I'd let her feel my purse.

Playing Dress-Up

Going beyond shoes and bags, vegans avoid animal-sourced textiles and discover other fascinating fabrics. There are plant fibers such as linen (which comes from flax), hemp, and cotton (organic cotton is particularly soft and luxurious). Versatile rayon, or viscose, sounds synthetic but it's a hybrid made from regenerated cellulose, the main constituent of plant cell walls. And today's microfibers and surprising new fabrics made from recycled materials can lead to a wardrobe that's lacking in nothing.

Most of the time, we'll purchase our "vegan" clothes, whether new, vintage, or thrift, at stores that stock other kinds of clothing, too. When you ask the clerk, "Is this wool?" and she answers, "Even better—cashmere," and you say, "Oh, that's too bad. I'm looking for a non-animal fabric," you're educating the sales associate that cruelty, even when it took place far away and out of sight, is not a selling point.

When my daughter, Adair, was in the Walk for Farm Animals, the NYC edition of an annual nationwide event benefitting Farm Sanctuary, she noticed a street vendor energetically hawking scarves and shawls with shouts of "Genuine pashmina, only $10." Pashmina, when it is indeed "genuine," is goat's wool. Seeing that his potential customers were carrying signs with animal rights messages, he changed his pitch to "Fake pashmina! No animals were harmed." Now, I don't sanction telling lies (although, in this case, I don't know if the lie was before he changed his spiel or after), but the message is clear that when someone in business knows what customers want, that's what they want to provide.

The foundation for cruelty-free fashion has been laid already by talented and vocal vegetarian and vegan designers. The most famous is probably Stella McCartney. Her designs include no fur or leather or even glue with animal ingredients, although she does use wool from sheep the company believes did not undergo mulesing. Fashion consultant Tim Gunn of *Project Runway* is a vegetarian and animal rights proponent. Designer John Bartlett (JohnBartlettNY.com) is a committed vegan in both his life and his collection, as is the already mentioned haberdashery hero Joshua Katcher, of BraveGentleMan.com.

Lois Eastlund (LoisEastlund.com) celebrates vegan style in handmade yet affordable dresses; they are contemporary with a nod to mod and they make any woman look amazing. Alabama Chanin (AlabamaChanin.com) makes every garment to order—each one vegan and eco-sensitive. Another of my personal favorites from the growing list of designers who are compelling a stubborn fashion establishment to take them seriously is Leanne Mai-ly Hilgart, the force of nature behind Vaute Couture (VauteCouture.com).

Leanne trained as an elementary school teacher and did a stint in modeling, but her heart was always with the animals. She looked around to see what was missing, where animals were being abused to provide some product for which no viable alternative existed. What she saw: winter coats. The frosty months had nearly everyone snuggling into wool, down, or, heaven forbid, fur. Other than fake fur or a canvas trench with lots of sweaters underneath, there weren't a lot of choices. (I know this; I made do with wool coats from secondhand stores back when *vintage* was just plain *old*.)

So Leanne came up with a warm, gorgeous, animal-free, eco-friendly, recycled material. She also hatched a plan to fund production by giving people on her newsletter list deep discounts for early ordering, generating the cash for the manufacture of that season's fabrics. She committed to making the coats themselves in the United States, paying people well, and expressing the fullness of being vegan—by not just being kind to animals and indifferent otherwise, but kind to animals, caring toward humans, and respectful of the environment; and she expressed all this through drop-dead, unbelievable, OMG-you've-gotta-see-these, gorgeous coats.

Then she diversified, as entrepreneurs tend to do, by creating other fabrics and discovering a way to do a down-free puffer coat toasty enough to brave Lake Shore winters in her native Chicago. And since it isn't always cold out (see: there is a God), she expanded into lighter-weight jackets for women and men, and pants, skirts, and the most adorable dresses, many of which have her signature open-star closure in the back.

Leanne and Vaute (you *vote* with your lifestyle choices for the kind of world you want) had the first ever show in New York City Fashion Week that was 100 percent vegan and cruelty free. Several of the models came out with dogs from the Humane Society and many of those canines on the catwalk got homes. While fashion magazines like to use animals of all sorts for their aesthetic contribution to a photo spread, this was compassion and fashion together for real. When you add those up, you know what you get? Beautiful.

Chloé Jo's Story

On my first date with Jeremy, he made it clear he was "okay" with my veganism, as long as I didn't try to turn him into a "namby-pamby vegetarian." He was a rock 'n' roll tough guy, covered in tattoos, and with the spirit and work ethic of a Jewish boy from Great Neck. He wanted no part in the stereotype of veganism. I was newly into veggie living myself. Raised on the Upper East Side of Manhattan, an impassioned socialite, carnivore, bon vivant, and party girl, I'd finally come to see my hypocritical love for my dogs but apparent contempt for all the other animals I ate (and wore) with zeal.

I did stop eating any animals or by-products except fish (!); I called myself a "pesco-vegan." I wasn't in a vegan community yet, nor did I stop wearing leather miniskirts (misguided '90s fashion choices). I had a copy of the animal agriculture documentary *Peaceable Kingdom* that I'd never watched. Still, I knew something in just the word "vegan" felt extremely right to me. A few dates in, I wanted to prove to Jeremy how wrong it was to eat animals, but the truth was, I wasn't yet able to articulate the multitudinous ways veganism was optimal for body, mind, spirit, planet, *and* animals. I was in need of an education. Under the guise of "Hey, I've seen this all before, but I'll watch it again with you," I brought my DVD of *Peaceable Kingdom* to Jeremy's fourth-floor walk-up apartment in the East Village.

Over a dinner of Chinese takeout, we watched the jaw-dropping truth bombs of what goes down in our "food" system. Jeremy moved away from me and asked to pause the documentary. He fell to the floor weeping. "I didn't know. I didn't know," he kept saying, followed by, "I will never eat an animal again." We both went vegan that day.

And I fell deeply in love. What sort of man cries for pigs and chickens? A real man, that's who.

And that day, two cynical Jew Yorkers came together as not only activists, but life partners. We were married shortly after and welcomed five rescued pets and three beautiful human vegan baby boys in close succession. Jeremy is my soul mate, but I believe our mission of kindness to animals keeps us connected and energetically intertwined. I know if I hadn't been on my veggie path, my heart would have been holding on to the blockages left by my less-than-stellar childhood and off-course prior romance decisions. Instead, I felt clear, open-eyed, ready for love—because I was so full of passion to help animals.

Jeremy and I were fated to meet (we found out much later that we'd actually met once as children, poolside at the

King David Hotel in Israel), and our mission keeps us full of love and blessings. I thank my lucky stars every day for the asteroid of clarity that allowed me to be brave enough to watch that film that particular day. This changed the trajectory of my life and business and led me to change my website, Girlie GirlArmy.com, from a fashion and nightlife hub to an encyclopedia of glam, green, vegan—and most important—ethical living.

I wanted to do vegan gorgeously and in my urban, glittery way, and I knew there must be others who eschewed hairy legs but still ate tofu. (Of course, now that I'm a mom of three under the age of five, I'm more lax on the hairy legs, but I still love sharing the news on sexy plant-based living daily with my thousands of longtime readers.)

All in all, following a mission of non-harming allows you to be focused enough to find your true love, and it allows you to love yourself in ways you never thought possible before. Having a laser-sharp set of scruples through which to see the world is the ultimate in true love. The muted way we can sometimes convince ourselves that someone is "the one" just isn't possible when you are living in full authenticity. We're raising our children to have respect for all living things, and our love story grows stronger every day.

—**Chloé Jo Davis**, mother, author, lifestyle expert, and activist. GirlieGirlArmy.com

24
......

The Body Electric

Walt Whitman includes in *Leaves of Grass* a poem called "I Sing the Body Electric." He writes, "If any thing is sacred, the human body is sacred . . . That of male is perfect and that of female is perfect." These are stark alternatives to "My thighs are disgusting."

His poem is generally regarded as a paean to sensuality, and on one level I suppose it is, but Whitman was also a mystic. This is the same man who wrote, "To me, every minute of light and dark is a miracle. Every cubic inch of space is a miracle." I believe that his term "body electric," has to do with not only attributes of the physical form but with that *otherness*, the spirit that infuses the body. I've observed that as people become more and more aware of this subtle, but perhaps truest, aspect of who they are, they gravitate toward different foods—lighter, brighter, more life, less death.

The first raw fooder I ever knew was a former Indiana steelworker who, back in the 1980s, hosted monthly vegetarian potlucks in Chicago, where I was living at the time. Those of us who came to be regulars would sometimes meet for dinner in between times, often at a Middle Eastern place offering falafel, hummus, and the like. This gentleman would have salad—not a big, interesting salad that even a lot of conventional restaurants offer nowadays, but a puny, pitiful 1980s salad made of iceberg lettuce with a pale tomato wedge.

I felt sorry for my raw friend at those dinners and thought he had willpower made of the same steel he had once forged at the mill. Today I see it differently. He was living in the body electric. He felt strong and balanced and in tune with himself. For him to have made an exception for white pita bread and a smear of baba ghanoush would have altered his vibratory level in a way that would have been unpleasant for him. Not eating falafel was no more difficult for him than it was for me not to eat cat food.

I should have understood that sooner. A yoga teacher had told me prophetically when I was only nineteen, "Don't bother changing your diet. Yoga will change your diet." It took some time, and in my case, the metamorphosis didn't come specifically from yoga, if you think of that in terms of headstand and downward-facing dog. But yoga, by definition, also means *union*, which did lead to my lifestyle change. As I became more unified—imperfectly, but better—with other people, other beings, and the Divine within, my food choices, and many other choices, changed, too.

Food and Spirit

Learning about the link between food and spirituality can be either illuminating or disconcerting to us Westerners because our culture sees the body as so, well, *physical*, and we have the idea that physicality and spirituality are polar opposites. This simply isn't so. In fact, as long as we're inhabiting a body, we cannot do spiritual practice, contemplate spiritual truths, or have a spiritual experience without its cooperation and participation.

Those who are blessed with this insight come to see that they are spiritual entities living in physical bodies, which are, in themselves, as remarkable as Whitman described. I saw this enunciated again on the business card of a Los Angeles acupuncturist who promised "insightful care of the precious physical envelope and the spirit within." When you look at washing your hair and shopping for groceries and going to the gym as ways to care for the "precious physical envelope," these otherwise mundane activities take on the importance they've long deserved.

This care doesn't call for elaborate rituals or exotic dishes. Many years ago, I heard the late Rukmini Devi Arundale, a noted Indian classical dancer, recount the story of being asked to a luncheon by Eleanor Roosevelt. The invitation had come at the end of a long U.S. tour and the diminutive dancer reluctantly prepared herself for one more heavy, multicourse meal. Instead, the First Lady chose a menu of cottage cheese and fresh fruit. Rukmini commented that this was her best meal in America.

Now, if you're a committed vegan, don't hate me (or Mrs. Roosevelt) for the part about cottage cheese. We're only responsible for what we know, and I'm sure that neither woman saw a moral compromise in her curds and whey. I didn't either, for the first many years of my life, and that's probably true for you, too. I tell this story merely to illustrate that simplicity, in food and in life, is a precious thing.

Just Desserts

The upshot of all this is that two wonderful, spiritual shifts take place after you've eaten a kind and colorful diet for a reasonable period of time. First comes the peace you'll feel when your survival no longer depends on someone else's death. Your body will find its own place of harmony once it's been freed from having to process decaying flesh and the bodily chemicals produced from pain and fear at the time of an animal's slaughter. You've heard of the sound sleep that comes with a clear conscience? Being vegan means sound sleep and clear thinking and more exuberance and greater peace. You will experience all of these, in one order or another. I'm not promising some fantasy life with no problems, but when clouds show up, their silver linings won't be so darned hard to get to.

GKT

Cocoa (or cacao, raw cocoa powder) is always vegan and most dark chocolate bars are, too (check the label). Substances in cocoa can reduce inflammation from sun exposure and increase circulation to the skin. Be sure you're buying ethical chocolate not harvested with slave labor. See *Vegan Chocolate*, by Fran Costigan, for more information.

Second, you'll have a subtle but sweet awareness of the body electric, that your physical energy is buoyed up by a spiritual energy you can't help but notice and can't begin to describe. The fresh foods you're eating will provide more than nutrients, more even than the phytochemicals that protect against disease. These foods are more than repositories of the best water you can put into your body, hydrating your skin and supporting the myriad water-dependent chemical reactions constantly taking place inside you.

Included in this "more," if you're willing to credit fruits and vegetables with something that can't be shown, at least not yet, via laboratory assay, is the invisible energy the yogis call *prana*. According to ancient teachings, this is what causes a seed to sprout or a flower to blossom. It only sounds woo-woo until you start to feel it and see it, when you wake up and can no longer lament looking bad in the mornings because you look really lovely. This is when you get the fabled "glow" and people start wondering what seductive secret you're holding close that's responsible for the uncanny radiance.

210 | The Good Karma Diet

How long will this take? It varies some from person to person, but I'll give you an approximation of three weeks to see the early glimmerings, six months for it to blossom brilliantly, and two years for the change to be cell-deep and soul-deep. When that happens, you won't feel that you're a different person exactly, but rather a more complete person than you were before. Is this a lot to expect from something so seemingly prosaic as a change in your diet? It isn't. I've been saying all along that this will get you good karma.

Deirdre's Good Karma Story

Starting a vegan lifestyle has brought me good karma tenfold. Before the switch I had no spirituality in my life. I didn't think anything happened for a reason and I felt disconnected from everything. I'm not sure exactly how it happened, but within weeks of becoming vegan, I started to feel more rooted to the earth. Great food became something that I really appreciated. I think when I had to pay attention to what I was consuming, I became aware of how lucky we all are to have food and life and choices.

I was also introduced to many amazing teachers: Kris Carr, Victoria Moran, and other like-minded, loving, strong vegans. These new influences really opened my eyes to living with gratitude, grace, and kindness. That immediately opened the door to what I could only call a positive karma flow. When you live gently and lovingly, you will be rewarded. People seem a bit nicer. Funny little "coincidences" that really help you out become almost commonplace. When all of these great little things started to happen, I couldn't help but take note. Everything in my world was changing. It was getting brighter, and I was getting more optimistic.

I'd already lost a lot of weight—over one hundred

pounds—and the final twenty-five came off after going vegan. Otherwise, that year was not what I would consider a great one—a lot of trials and tribulations, as we all have at times in our lives. The difference between that year and other wacky years, though, was that this time I wasn't so worried about it. There was this sense that I was going to be okay, that everything would work out in the most perfect way. And you know what? It did. And it helped me grow into a better, more compassionate woman.

A vegan way of life, simply put, opened up something in my heart that allowed me access to a deep spirituality I never knew I had. Once that happened—boom! Instant karma. And why not? A life of immense love and gratitude can only bring positive energy—to you and everyone around you.

What I know for sure today is that everything in life changes. People come and go; rules are altered and things come up. With love in your heart and compassion front and center, you can handle all of it with grace.

—**Deirdre "DeDe" Gaffke**, blogger, student of
the world. MidwestVibes.com

25
......

The Good Karma Life

People eat in all kinds of ways for all kinds of reasons. Most of the time, food choices are reflexive, without a lot of thought behind them. Sometimes, however, we set out to get our act together. We eat more intentionally and, for a while anyway, we feel better. The changes are often short-lived. As anthropologist Margaret Mead astutely observed, "It's easier to change a man's religion than to change his diet." What most sets apart a Good Karma approach from the endless array of diets that sell books and spawn products and become part of the cultural vernacular is that it affords anyone who approaches it with sincerity a deeply satisfying way of being in the world.

GKT

When dining out, read between the lines. If you're with clients at a steakhouse and the menu has Caesar salad (with anchovies and raw egg), you know there's romaine lettuce in the kitchen. If the steaks come with a baked potato and vegetable *du jour*, you can have veggies on your salad and a spud or two on the side. Ask for no butter and top your tater with A.1. steak sauce, Heinz 57, mustard, or a drizzle of olive oil.

In a Good Karma Life, the spontaneous joy you feel from having a body that's functioning as well as it can joins with the deep satisfaction of knowing that, even though you can't make everything perfect, you're making a heck of a lot of things better. A veganward revision of your food choices does this in a way no other lifestyle alteration can. No other action simultaneously benefits your body, other creatures, and the entire living, breathing ecosystem. And it's so easy: you were going to make dinner anyway.

Sometimes people embark on this way of eating, this way of living, as almost a dare: "All right, show me you're better than the diet I did last year or the one I'll try next if you don't work." That is not an attitude conducive to success. Here's one that is: "My heart is telling me to do this, and if everything about it doesn't suit me seamlessly right away, I'm willing to do some troubleshooting until it does." That troubleshooting may consist of trying some different foods or food combinations, expanding your culinary repertoire, making friends with other vegans, or enlisting the services of a vegan lifestyle coach or a knowledgeable health care professional. You know from past experience that when the will is there, the way presents itself. My intention in writing this book is to give you "grist for the will," as it were, sufficient information and motivation so that you're committed to take it from here. "Go forth and set the world on fire," Saint Ignatius told his students. We can still do that.

GKT

Make life easy at restaurants. You know those little return-address labels you can order for a couple dollars? There's no law that an address has to be printed on them. You might try: "No meat, poultry, fish, eggs, or dairy products—nothing from an animal, all vegan please—thank you." The server

Go out, then, as a force for good in a world that's imprecise and uncertain. It's fantastic if your grandmother is eating vegan, even if the orthopedic shoes she needs to wear come only in leather. It's wonderful that your pooch is thriving on his vegetarian kibble, even though your cat eats meat. When enough people are vegan, every kind of shoe will be, too. When the "cloned meats" are perfected and widely available—check out ModernMeadow.com—Kitty can eat the food she needs without limiting anybody else's life. We have a way to go on all this, but we've come a long way, too.

Begin with one recipe, one meal, or one exploratory tour of your grocery store. It's like the long journey that starts with the first step, except this one starts with the first bite. Eat plants, favor fresh, and go "as raw as you wanna be," a phrase I learned from Bob Dagger, founder of High Vibe market in NYC (HighVibe.com). He's a mentor of mine and you'll want to have one, or several, yourself—in person or on YouTube or wherever you can access their wisdom.

If you're just starting out, your family will go through a transition period that is likely to be more difficult than your own. You've embarked on an incredible journey. If you were going on an adventure vacation, you'd probably be so filled with excitement that worry would have no place to land. It's those left behind who'd fret about your health and safety and whether you'd packed enough of everything. As you make this adventurous change in your diet, negotiate kindly and clearly with the people you live with and your extended family. Your mom won't really die of a broken heart because you don't taste the turkey at Thanksgiving, and "mixed marriages" can work just fine—there's a whole book on the subject, in fact: *Kitchen Divided*, by Ellen Jaffe Jones.

The most important things for the people who love you are that you'll still be you and that they can still be who they are. Reassurance on these fronts goes a long way. Be cheerful and tolerant and stick to your guns. Bring your most delectable dishes to share at family gatherings—and to the office, for that matter. Have the recipe printed up if someone wants a copy, but don't harp about its being vegan. "Yummy" speaks volumes.

We started this book with my Good Karma story. In the time that's passed since I wrote that, I realize even more that everything I dreamed of as an awkward kid has become and continues to morph into the reality of my life. Of course I experience challenges and annoyances and disappointments like everybody else, but the bright spots are so bright, I'm ceaselessly amazed.

Not long ago, for example, the editors of the online magazine *La Fashionista Compassionista* came to my place with their photographer, Chris Pearce (a great-looking guy with an English accent. I needed to tell you that to give you more of the effect). They put me in gorgeous clothes and took pictures for the publication. Now, I've told you that I'm sixty-four, and that when I was young and thought fashion models were goddesses incarnate, I was struggling with acne and my weight and subterranean self-esteem. That Saturday in my apartment with the dresses and accessories and photographic equipment, the impossible dream of my earlier life took shape before my eyes.

There's a beautiful quotation in the biblical book of Joel: "I will give you the years the locust has eaten." I discovered that passage when I'd been free from compulsive overeating and dieting and hating the way I looked just long enough to believe it could stick. When I read those words, I felt an immediate affinity: I was getting back lost time. I felt the same way at that photo shoot. I know I'm not going to go out and be some senior-citizen supermodel, but I had the *experience* of that. And it was sublime.

I can't tell you for certain how much my vegan principles have to do with all this "good karma," but I can pinpoint the day that things picked up and sped up and the dreams-come-true machine went into overdrive. It was the day I decided to focus the rest of my life on helping animals be happier and people be healthier. Most people who stop eating animals and start eating plants won't make a career of it, but virtually everyone I know who has simply changed their food choices in this way finds that everything in their lives picks up: career, creativity, energy, serendipity, joy.

Sometimes, when first confronted with the suffering of the animals and the plight of the planet, a new vegan goes through a period of depression—"How can something this horrific be going on?"—or anger—"How can you claim to be a good person and keep on eating animals?"—or both. These are natural reactions and not unjustified. The only problem is, they don't help.

Changing what you eat is the first step—the easy one. Then you have to open your heart—not just the physical arteries that we know can open on this kind of diet, but the metaphorical heart, the one that can draw in enough compassion for animals and people, too. The superior food you're eating will nourish you, but that love will sustain you. It will keep you on track and give you the most glorious gifts: the ability to effect positive change in the world, and the grace not to measure the scope of your influence but simply be grateful to have some.

If you read this book because you wanted to lose weight, or ease an irritating tummy issue, or get your doctor off your back about your cholesterol or blood pressure or something else, I trust that your scale and your stomach and your GP will be giving you a thumbs-up before you know it. I also happen to believe there are no accidents. The way life operates, from my point of view, is that you got hold of this book instead of some other one because your soul is as ready to expand as your body is to heal.

Something is going on here that's bigger and grander than either of us and everybody's doctor besides. Human history has been a saga of man against nature, and might being right. What if we're on the threshold of something revolutionary? What if our evolution is about to shift in favor of cooperation with nature, respect for all beings, and harnessing the power of love? What if you and I and our daily choices could be a vital part of bringing this about? I can't think of anything more exciting. So what do you say? Shall we do this? Start—slowly if you need to, but start just the same. And when you have one, I'd love to hear your Good Karma story.

Appendix A

......

Life Can Be Hard, So Food Should Be Easy Recipes

—Doris Fin, CHHC, AADP

first met Victoria virtually through the "Creating a Charmed Life" lecture she presented at the school I attended, the Institute for Integrative Nutrition, and in person a few months later at Veggie Fest Hamilton, in Ontario. Since I felt as if I already knew her, I eagerly shared with her images of dozens of raw dishes I'd conceived and developed. When she asked if I'd be interested in writing the recipes for this book, with its all-plant and high-raw but not all-raw philosophy, it felt like a perfect collaboration: different generations, similar food philosophy, and a shared passion for changing this world for the better.

The way I look at recipes is that, like rules, you either follow them to the letter—that can provide some reassurance if you're new to the culinary arts, or to this type of cuisine—or you can allow them to be suggestions on which you can improvise to suit your palate and the rhythm of your life. I enjoy a variety of tastes, textures, and, most important, colors. Infused with the most exquisite of these, raw food has been the greatest treasure for creativity in my kitchen.

Each recipe I'm offering you here was inspired by my travels around the world—and I have a decided preference for destinations that are off the beaten path. One of the rewards of wanderlust is waking up in sight of nutritious foods such as maca, quinoa, cacao, various seeds and nuts, avocado, olives, and other fruits growing right before my eyes. Coming to know these foods in their natural habitat—really "getting it" that cacao is a bean long before it's a chocolate bar—whet my desire to play with their endless potential.

Before we get to the recipes, there are a few notes I would like to share to make the planning and prep behind Good Karma dining a little easier—and a lot of fun. First: Refuse to be intimidated by any recipe you see anywhere. When you're working with fresh fruits and vegetables, they're complete in themselves. Cooking and other preparation is really just accessorizing what nature has already perfected. When you are using a recipe, take comfort in knowing that plant-based dishes in general, and raw cuisine in particular, seldom require strict adherence, so there's some room for you to improvise and experiment.

Vegetables: These are mainstays of a high-raw, whole-food diet. Wherever vegetables are required, call on an understudy when you need to. Substituting one leafy green for another, or a different root veggie for one of those in the recipe, will create a slightly different dish. Ditto for adding more or less of a particular ingredient.

Potatoes: To retain their nutrients and flavor, it's best to steam potatoes, unpeeled, rather than boil or bake them. There are many varieties of potatoes, so experiment with different kinds. Try sweet potatoes, and the pink, purple, red, yellow, and brown varieties of the familiar spud; the external skin color rarely affects the inside hue. If you're sugar-sensitive, sweet potatoes are actually a better choice for you than white. Buy organic whenever possible: conventional potatoes can be heavily sprayed. Organic tastes better, and this kind of farming is kinder to the earth.

Fruit: When a recipe calls for fruit, you can often use a different one, especially if you stay in the same family, e.g., an orange for a tangerine, an apple for a pear, cantaloupe for honeydew. Avoid mixing melons with other fruit as they digest more quickly and may interfere with the digestion of other foods if eaten with them.

Freezing bananas: A frozen banana is the key to a creamy, soda-fountain-style smoothie. To freeze bananas, be sure they're ripe (wait till they have some brown speckles) but catch them before they feel soft. Peel the bananas, cut into 1-inch pieces, and freeze in an airtight plastic bag or other airtight container. In a good freezer with a consistent 0°F temperature, they'll last up to three weeks.

Non-dairy milks: When a recipe calls for non-dairy milk, you can use homemade nut milk (I'll give you a recipe for a basic Brazil nut or almond milk you can use in smoothies, on cereals, and for most other purposes) or commercial plant milk—soy, almond, rice, oat, hemp, coconut, etc. Always buy the unsweetened variety, and if you're going with soy, be sure the carton says either "organic" or "non-GMO," since most soy is genetically modified.

Spices and culinary herbs: Try them all. Use organic when possible to obtain optimal nutrient density and richer flavor. The better the quality of the herb or spice, the more likely it's been less treated, less processed, and less heated. Check the expiration date (and the manufacture and packing dates, if available), and unless you're buying organic from a trusted brand such as Frontier Herbs, be sure the label says "non-irradiated." Otherwise, the product has likely been treated with ionizing radiation; the rationale is to kill bacteria, but the result is an herb or spice lacking many of its beneficial properties.

Dry your own herbs when possible, and store all herbs and spices in airtight containers, preferably glass. Avoid direct sunlight or heat. You can buy spices whole and grind them yourself—they're cheaper and fresher, and grinding brings out full-on flavor; if you purchase dried and powdered herbs and spices, buy them in small quantities and freeze those you don't use often (holiday-season spices, for instance).

In the recipes that follow, measures are given for dried spices unless fresh is indicated. And here's a tip of the raw food trade: using garlic powder and onion powder can give raw dishes a more "cooked" or "complete" mouthfeel. When using fresh garlic, note that it's far more pungent raw than cooked, so start with quite a bit less for a raw dish than you'd use in a cooked one.

Cinnamon: Conventional cinnamon can contain a naturally occurring carcinogenic compound. This is probably nothing to worry about when you're using the spice only in recipes, but if you want to include cinnamon in your smoothies, oatmeal, puddings, etc., on a regular basis to benefit from its high antioxidant content, purchase Ceylon cinnamon. It's a different strain of the plant and does not include the questionable compound.

Sweeteners: Maple syrup, brown rice syrup, molasses, and agave can stand in for one another in equivalent amounts. Non-caloric stevia is some ten times sweeter than sugar and getting a bit too much means a taste of bitter with the sweet, so use only a few drops (if liquid) or a careful measure (if powdered). Each sweetener has its own distinct characteristics, so experiment with different ones to discover which suits you and your creation most.

Raw dessert recipes often call for dates, providing sweetness from a whole food. ("Date sugar" is just ground dried dates, so it's also a whole-food sweetener that can substitute, measure for measure, for brown sugar in a recipe; granulated coconut sugar can do this, too.) Medjool dates are the plumpest and most tender variety, but if they're unavailable, or they're out of your price range, you can work with any dates. Those that feel very dry and hard will benefit from thirty minutes' soaking in pure water.

Vanilla: Often from exotic locales such as Madagascar, Tahiti, or Thailand, this tropical climbing orchid produces pods containing vanilla beans, source of the familiar fragrance and flavor. You can purchase the pods, cut them open, and scrape out the beans inside, or buy pre-dried powder. If you like using vanilla extract, look to a company such as Simply Organic that uses no preservatives, sweeteners, or artificial flavorings. Where the recipe calls for ¼ teaspoon of fresh vanilla bean, you can substitute 1 teaspoon of vanilla extract.

Salt: I personally never use iodized or refined salt, and recommend instead Celtic and Himalayan salts, which come from cleaner sources and have their naturally occurring minerals intact. If you follow my lead on this, or if for your own reasons you avoid salt entirely, be sure you're eating seaweeds or otherwise meeting your requirements for iodine.

Raw nuts and seeds: Soaking nuts is important to deactivate the enzyme inhibitors in them; it also makes them easier to digest and increases their volume. Different nuts call for different soaking times, and raw food chefs differ in their preferred soaking times. I generally soak raw cashews, walnuts, and macadamias for 4 to 6 hours; harder nuts, such as almonds, filberts, or Brazils, can soak for up to 8 hours. These are approximate times; any soaking is better than none, unless a specific recipe, such as for a raw cake or piecrust, specifies unsoaked nuts.

If a recipe calls for a nut you don't have on hand, use a similar one, i.e., raw cashews to replace macadamias, or pecans to stand in for walnuts. Store nuts in containers in the fridge or freezer; refrigeration is all the more important if nuts have been ground or chopped. Soaked nuts keep refrigerated for up to five days. Keep all nuts and seeds out of direct sunlight and check packaging dates to assure freshness. (A note on hempseeds: technically, hempseeds are in their shells; hemp *hearts* are hulled. When a recipe calls for hempseeds, I'm referring to hulled seeds or hearts.)

Roasted nuts and seeds: Avoid buying pre-roasted nuts and seeds as they tend to be heated at high temperatures and may be rancid by the time you buy them. If you like the toasty taste, do it yourself. Heat a dry skillet over medium heat (cast iron works beautifully for this), add the raw nuts (not too many), and stir continuously with a wooden spoon until the nuts are slightly browned; remove them from the pan immediately. This is a quick task—small seeds, such as sunflower, roast in almost no time; larger nuts will take longer.

Coconut: Victoria and I agree to disagree when it comes to coconut. My contention is that the medium-chain fatty acids in coconut metabolize differently from other saturated fats (i.e., animal fats and palm oil), and the healing benefits of coconut and coconut oil are widely documented. My colleague holds to the more conventional view that a sat fat is a sat fat, to be used sparingly, if at all, especially by anyone with a history (or family history) of heart disease or high cholesterol. I keep dried, unsweetened, whole coconut in my kitchen; Victoria would use dried, unsweetened, fat-reduced coconut—the same flavor and texture without the fat. I also use coconut oil (more on oils below) for some food prep, while Victoria uses this rich fat mostly for cosmetic application, or perhaps in a very special dessert on some rare occasion.

Oils: When one of these recipes calls for olive oil, I'm trusting that you'll use cold-pressed, extra-virgin olive oil, organic if possible. You can keep coconut and olive oil in your pantry; if you use the more delicate oils that break down rapidly—hempseed or flaxseed oil— keep them refrigerated and never use them past the expiry date.

Preservatives and additives: When purchasing packaged products, read the ingredients carefully. Look out for preservatives and words you cannot pronounce, usually artificial substances put in to prolong shelf life or add unnatural color. Lemon juice and salt are natural preservatives, and including one or both of these in some of the recipes that follow enables them to last longer in the fridge.

Organic foods: Choose organic whenever possible, both for your own health and to support superior agriculture. (There may also be small farms in your area that are virtually organic but can't afford the high cost of organic certification. Talk with the farmers and find out how they do things.) When you buy conventional produce, peel these fruits and veggies when possible and wash them well, perhaps adding a bit of distilled white vinegar to the water.

Chopping: The smaller the cut, the more flavor is released—for example, minced garlic has more intensity than coarsely chopped or whole garlic. On the other hand, finely chopped, diced, minced, or shredded foods, as well as any dish prepared with a blender or food processor, oxidize more rapidly, so plan to eat these freshly prepared or within a day or two, unless otherwise stated in the recipe.

Resources: Two of my favorite superfood and health food companies, whose products are widely available in health food stores as well as online, are Giddy Yoyo (GiddyYoyo.com) and Sunfood Superfoods (SunFood.com). Among the ingredients I access from these sources are Tahitian vanilla powder, raw fair-trade cacao powder, mesquite powder, and green powders for smoothies. Just reading the websites of companies like these can be an education. When you see an ingredient with which you're unfamiliar in a smoothie recipe or elsewhere, do a quick search and see if it looks like something you'd like to try. Most of the time, what you're making will be plenty "super," even without the more exotic additions.

Loving preparation: You'll see that the instructions for every recipe bear the notation "Loving Preparation." I believe this is at least as important to the dish you're making as the quality of its ingredients. If you were lucky enough to remember dishes prepared by a mother or grandmother who often cooked from scratch and took pride in feeding her family as well as she knew how, you already know that love imparts something to a dish that even the finest imported spices can't. You're choosing Good Karma foods, fresh and whole and kind; preparing them lovingly brings the good karma full circle.

Life in the Juice Lane

Freshly squeezed juices, with an emphasis on vegetables and greens, are key players in a high-raw diet. They provide concentrated nutrition and have the uncanny ability to encourage the person enjoying them to want to consume simpler, fresher foods. Sometimes cutting down on junk food can be as easy as adding a 16-ounce glass of juice to your day, either first thing in the morning, at that sluggish point in mid-afternoon, or as a before-dinner vitality cocktail.

Green Dreams

....

INGREDIENTS:

INGREDIENTS:

2 medium green apples

1 medium field cucumber

6 medium stalks celery

1 handful fresh parsley, with stems

2 tablespoons freshly squeezed lemon juice

LOVING PREPARATION:

1. Rinse all the veggies and fruits.
2. Slice the apples and cucumber so they fit into the juicer.
3. Juice all the ingredients except the lemon juice and strain.
4. Stir in the lemon juice and drink immediately.

NOTE To add extra coolness to this or any fresh juice, add a couple of ice cubes.

Makes about 16 ounces

Beet the Competition

....

INGREDIENTS:

1 medium beet

1 medium field cucumber

6 medium stalks celery

1 (2-inch) piece fresh ginger

½ cup pineapple chunks

2 tablespoons freshly squeezed lemon juice

LOVING PREPARATION:

1. Rinse all the veggies.
2. Slice the beet and cucumber so they fit into the juicer.
3. Juice all the ingredients except the lemon juice and strain.
4. Stir in the lemon juice and drink immediately.

Makes about 16 ounces

Beauty and the Brunch

. . . .

INGREDIENTS:

2 fennel stalks

1 medium field cucumber

6 medium stalks celery

1 medium green apple

10 strawberries, with leaves

1 handful fresh mint, with stems

1 tablespoon freshly squeezed lemon juice

LOVING PREPARATION:

1. Rinse all the veggies, fruit, and the mint. To clean the fennel, cut off the base of the bulb so it is easy to peel off the stalks and rinse them.

2. Slice the cucumber, fennel, and apple so they fit into the juicer.
3. Juice all the ingredients except the lemon juice and strain.
4. Stir in the lemon juice and drink immediately.

Makes about 16 ounces

Good Morning, Good Karma

When people start to eat more whole plant foods, they're sometimes stumped about breakfast. With such standbys as bacon and eggs, most boxed cereals, dairy yogurt, and breakfast pastries out of the picture, there needs to be a revamp of the morning meal. With just a little shift in your thinking, this can be as easy as it is delicious. Fruits, nuts and nut butters, and whole grains are a.m. naturals, and the advent of the green smoothie has invited those super-healthy leafy greens to show up for breakfast, too.

Brazil Nut Milk
. . . .

INGREDIENTS:

1 cup Brazil nuts (or almonds), soaked in water for 6 hours or
   overnight, rinsed, and drained
4 cups water
⅛ teaspoon good-quality salt, such as Himalayan pink salt
   (recommended wherever salt is used)
1 tablespoon maple syrup (optional)
¼ teaspoon vanilla bean powder, or 1 teaspoon vanilla extract
   (optional)

1. Blend the nuts in 1 cup of the water in a blender until the water becomes white and the nuts are completely pulverized.
2. Add the rest of the water and the remaining ingredients.
3. Although the milk can be used as is for smoothies, to get a smooth beverage for drinking, strain and squeeze the milk through a nut milk bag or sprouting bag. (You can find these at a natural food store or order online from HighVibe.com or any retailer appealing to the raw food market.) If you don't have one on hand, you can use a fine-mesh strainer, or line a coarser strainer with cheesecloth to extract the liquid from the nut pulp. Serve this nut milk hot or cold, sprinkled with cinnamon or cacao, if you like; or use on cereal or in a recipe just as you would dairy milk. The nut milk can be stored in a glass jar in the refrigerator for up to 7 days.

OPTIONS

Substitute 8 to 10 drops of liquid stevia for the maple syrup.

Add ½ teaspoon ground cinnamon.

Add 1 tablespoon raw fair-trade cacao powder to make a yummy chocolate milk you can even freeze into ice pops.

Makes 1 quart

Super-Spa Muesli

....

INGREDIENTS:

2½ cups rolled oats, uncooked

¼ cup hempseeds

¼ cup ground flaxseeds

¼ cup chopped dried fruit (currants, apricots, raisins, goji berries, etc., unsulfured and without oil)

¼ cup pumpkin seeds or sunflower seeds

¼ cup chopped almonds, walnuts, or hazelnuts

¼ teaspoon salt

½ teaspoon fresh vanilla bean powder

½ to 1 teaspoon ground cinnamon

For serving:

Water or non-dairy milk

Fresh berries

LOVING PREPARATION:

1. In a large bowl, mix together by hand, really well, the oats, hemp, flax, dried fruit, seeds, almonds, salt, vanilla, and cinnamon. Store in an airtight container or zipper bag in the refrigerator to retain its freshness.

2. To prepare 1 serving: Combine ½ cup muesli and 1 cup water or non-dairy milk in a jar or bowl. Soak overnight in the fridge (or, if using water, at room temperature). The muesli will soak up the liquid and expand in volume.

3. Serve with fresh berries, and more milk if you like.

Makes approximately 5 cups dry muesli. If single servings are prepared as directed, the yield is 10 servings.

Chia Seed Pudding

· · · · · · · ·

INGREDIENTS:

1 cup unsweetened non-dairy milk (homemade or
   commercial)
3 tablespoons chia seeds (whole or ground)
4 or 5 drops stevia, or 1 teaspoon maple syrup
½ teaspoon ground cinnamon
⅛ teaspoon vanilla bean powder, or ½ teaspoon vanilla extract

OPTIONAL:

1 tablespoon pumpkin seeds, sunflower seeds, or hempseeds
1 tablespoon chopped nuts
½ to 1 cup fresh berries of your choice

LOVING PREPARATION:

1. Stir together the milk, chia seeds, sweetener, cinnamon, and
   vanilla bean powder in a jar. Cover with a tight-fitting lid and let
   stand for 5 minutes.
2. After 5 minutes, shake the jar really well. Let stand for 5 minutes
   more, then shake really well again.
3. Let stand at room temperature for at least 20 minutes or, for best
   digestion, refrigerate overnight and serve for breakfast. You can
   also prepare this in the morning and leave it in the fridge for a
   midday or evening snack.
4. Before opening, shake vigorously one more time. Then pour into
   a bowl and add any or all of the optional ingredients.

Serves 2

Berry Brainy Smoothie

....

INGREDIENTS:

- 1 cup vegan milk of your choice
- ½ cup blueberries or mixed berries (fresh or frozen)
- 1 frozen banana
- 1 tablespoon hempseeds
- 1 tablespoon ground flaxseeds
- ½ teaspoon ground cinnamon
- 2 or 3 drops stevia, or 1 teaspoon maple syrup (optional)

LOVING PREPARATION:

1. Put all the ingredients in a blender and blend until smooth and creamy.

Serves 1 (double the ingredients to serve 2)

Elvis Smoothie

....

INGREDIENTS:

- 1 cup homemade nut milk or unsweetened commercial vegan milk
- 1 tablespoon unsalted and unsweetened peanut butter or almond butter
- 1 tablespoon cocoa powder (ideally, raw fair-trade cacao)

4 drops stevia, 1 teaspoon maple syrup, or 2 teaspoons
blackstrap molasses

1 or 2 frozen bananas

OPTIONAL:

1 scoop rice, hemp, Brazil nut, or other high-quality vegan
protein powder—plain, vanilla, or chocolate

LOVING PREPARATION:

1. Put all the ingredients in a blender and blend until smooth and
   creamy. Throw in a couple of ice cubes if you like it cooler and
   with more froth.
2. Pour into a glass and serve with a sprinkle of cacao powder.

Serves 1 (double the ingredients to serve 2)

Green Power Smoothie
· · · · · · · ·

INGREDIENTS:

1 large stalk celery, chopped

1 frozen banana, or ½ cup other frozen fruit (peaches,
pineapple, berries, etc.)

1 tablespoon freshly squeezed lemon juice

1 to 1½ cups water

About 1 cup tightly packed kale or spinach

For a greener smoothie: 1 to 2 teaspoons spirulina or barley grass powder, and/or a handful of fresh cilantro or parsley

For a sweeter smoothie: 1 teaspoon maple syrup, or 3 or 4 drops stevia

For a heftier smoothie: ½ small avocado, and/or 1 scoop vegan protein powder

For a spicy smoothie: 1 (½-inch) knob fresh ginger, or ⅛ teaspoon cayenne pepper

LOVING PREPARATION:

1. In a blender, blend the celery, banana, lemon juice, water, and any optional ingredients until liquefied.
2. Add the greens of your choice and blend until completely liquefied. Taste and adjust if necessary. (Go easy on the greens at first. The time will come when you'll fill the blender with them.)
3. Serve immediately.

Serves 1 to 2

Greeña Colada

· · · · · · · ·

INGREDIENTS:

1 cup coconut water

1 cup frozen pineapple chunks (see note)

1 ripe banana, fresh or frozen

1 to 2 cups fresh spinach

OPTIONAL:

For a richer shake: use coconut milk (from the carton, not canned) to replace coconut water

For a lighter drink: eliminate the banana and toss in a handful of ice cubes instead

Slice of fresh pineapple, for serving

LOVING PREPARATION:

1. Put all the ingredients in a blender and blend until smooth and creamy.
2. Serve in a tall glass with a slice of fresh pineapple.

NOTE If you don't have frozen pineapple, use ¾ cup fresh pineapple chunks and ¼ cup ice cubes.

Serves 2 to 3

The Soup Course

Nothing opens up the world of whole, plant cuisine as swiftly as soups. They're virtually foolproof and you can shift the seasonings until your soup is custom-made. Raw soups are so smooth and delicious that people who want to eat more raw food, but aren't yet big fans of salads and juices, can start this way. And when the winds of winter blow, there's no competition for a hot pot of simmering soup to warm you through and through.

Lean Green Cream Soup

....

1 medium tomato, chopped, or 10 cherry tomatoes

1 small clove garlic, chopped

1 medium stalk celery, chopped

1 tablespoon chopped fresh cilantro or parsley

1 small cucumber, chopped

1 cup water, room temperature or cool (see note for warm
variation)

½ teaspoon salt (or to taste)

¼ teaspoon ground turmeric

¼ teaspoon ground cumin

¼ to ½ teaspoon cracked black pepper or cayenne pepper
(optional)

1 medium avocado, pitted

GARNISH:

¼ cup nori seaweed strips (sheets cut into strips/squares),
or 1 teaspoon dulse/kelp flakes

2 tablespoons hempseeds

LOVING PREPARATION:

1. Put all the ingredients except the avocado and garnishes in a
blender and blend until creamy and smooth.
2. Add the avocado and blend briefly, just until mixed in.
3. To serve, pour the soup into individual bowls, divide the garnish
ingredients evenly among the bowls, and sprinkle over each

bowl of soup. Keep leftovers in an airtight glass jar in the refrigerator for up to 3 days.

NOTE For a slightly warmer version, use hot water (not boiling) or, if you have a high-speed blender such as a Vitamix, you can blend all the ingredients except the avocado long enough to heat the soup slightly and then add the avocado and garnishes.

Serves 3 to 4

You Say Tomah-To Soup
· · · · · · · ·

INGREDIENTS:

3 medium field tomatoes, chopped

½ cup sun-dried tomatoes, unsulfured, soaked in water for
1 hour

2 medium stalks celery, leaves intact, chopped

1 teaspoon dried tarragon

1 teaspoon dried oregano

½ teaspoon ground turmeric

1 tablespoon raw unfiltered apple cider vinegar or balsamic
vinegar

5 pitted dates, or 2 teaspoons maple syrup

2 small cloves garlic, chopped

¼ teaspoon cracked black pepper

2 cups water

½ teaspoon Himalayan or Celtic salt (only if tomatoes weren't preserved in salt)

½ teaspoon cayenne pepper, or 1 small chile pepper, seeded

GARNISH:

4 to 6 tablespoons sprouts (mung bean, lentil, clover, sunflower seed, etc.)

4 to 6 tablespoons finely chopped fresh cilantro, parsley, or scallions

LOVING PREPARATION:

1. Put all the ingredients in a blender and blend on high speed until liquefied and completely smooth.
2. Pour the soup into individual bowls and garnish as desired.

Makes 6 cups

Esau Was onto Something Lentil Soup
....

INGREDIENTS:

1 cup lentils, soaked overnight in 4 cups water, rinsed, and drained

2 medium onions: 1 whole and unpeeled, 1 peeled and thinly sliced

5 cups boiling water

2 tablespoons olive oil, or ½ cup water, for sautéing

2 small stalks celery, chopped

1 medium carrot, chopped or sliced

2 teaspoons salt (or to taste)

½ teaspoon ground turmeric

1 or 2 small cloves garlic, minced

1 tablespoon grated fresh ginger

OPTIONAL:

For a spicy variation: ¼ to ½ teaspoon cayenne pepper or chili powder

GARNISH:

2 tablespoons chopped fresh cilantro, parsley, or dill

3 tablespoons pumpkin or sunflower seeds

1 cup sprouts (mung bean, lentil, clover, sunflower seed, etc.)

LOVING PREPARATION:

1. Add the lentils and whole onion to the boiling water in a soup pot.
2. Return to a boil, cover, reduce the heat to low, and simmer for 20 minutes.
3. Meanwhile, sauté the sliced onion in the olive oil or water for 12 minutes over medium-low heat; keep covered and stir occasionally.
4. Add the celery and carrot to the soup, close the lid, remove from the heat, and let stand for 5 minutes.
5. Remove the whole onion from the pot and carefully peel it (the skin should come off easily).
6. Drain half the contents and add the solid content to a heatproof food processor or blender, along with the peeled onion, salt, and seasonings. Purée until smooth and creamy. (*Be very careful when blending hot liquids, as the sudden release of steam has a*

tendency to blow the lid off blenders. Be sure the lid is firmly in place and cover the lid with a towel for extra safety. Start the blender at its lowest speed, increasing it slowly.)

7. Transfer the pureed and drained liquid back to the pot, along with the sautéed onions, and stir well. You should have a half-creamy, half-chunky soup.

8. To serve, pour the soup into individual bowls and divide the garnish ingredients among them.

CREAMY VARIATION

For a cream of lentil soup, blend all the ingredients.

MUSHROOM VARIATION

When sautéing the onion, add 2 cups chopped fresh mushrooms, any variety, and sauté for an extra 10 minutes, covered, stirring occasionally. If using dried mushrooms, soak for at least 30 minutes before adding to the sauté. Shiitake, oyster, and morel mushrooms work really well with this recipe.

Makes 7 cups

Creamy Golden Squash Soup

· · · · · · · ·

INGREDIENTS:

6 cups boiling water

1 medium white onion, whole, unpeeled

1 medium butternut or walnut squash, cubed

1 small zucchini, cubed

1 medium carrot, peeled and chopped

1 medium red onion, sliced

2 tablespoons olive oil

1 medium stalk celery, chopped

1 tablespoon salt (or to taste)

½ teaspoon ground turmeric (or to taste)

2 teaspoons ground cumin (or to taste)

1 or 2 cloves garlic, chopped

½ teaspoon cracked black pepper (or to taste)

½ teaspoon ground cinnamon (or to taste)

½ cup walnuts, chopped and lightly toasted

GARNISH:

Parsley or cilantro sprigs

LOVING PREPARATION:

1. In a medium pot, combine the water, whole white onion, and squash. Bring to a boil, then simmer for 10 minutes.
2. Add the zucchini and carrot and simmer for 10 minutes more.
3. Meanwhile, sauté the sliced red onion in the olive oil over medium heat until golden brown. Set aside.
4. Drain the soup into a large bowl and set the liquid aside.
5. Discard the onion peel and put the peeled white onion, along with the drained soup ingredients, in a heatproof food processor or blender. Add the celery, salt, and all seasonings and purée until smooth and creamy. *(Be very careful when blending hot liquids as the sudden release of steam has a tendency to blow the lid off blenders. Be sure the lid is firmly in place and cover the lid with a towel for extra safety. Start the blender at its lowest speed, increasing it slowly.)*
6. Pour the blender contents back into the pot and add the drained stock and sautéed onions.

7. Adjust the flavor, if needed, with more salt, pepper, or any of the spices.

8. Serve hot or chilled, in bowls or mugs. Sprinkle with toasted walnuts and decorate with a sprig of parsley or cilantro.

9. Store the soup in an airtight container in the refrigerator for up to 3 days, or freeze in a plastic container or sealed BPA-free zipper bag.

NOTE If toasting your own chopped raw walnuts, toast in a dry skillet over medium heat for 5 minutes, stirring continuously, until lightly toasted. Remove from the heat immediately. You can also use this technique for toasting walnuts in the later recipe for Waldorf salad (One Wondrous Waldorf, page 247) and wherever you'd welcome a toasty crunch. Or, for a raw, easily digestible version, nuts can be soaked overnight, rinsed, drained, and dried on a paper towel for 30 minutes, then coarsely chopped.

"MEATY" VARIATION

If you love mushrooms and want a bit of a meaty texture, sauté 1 cup fresh or 10 soaked and sliced dried shiitake mushrooms with the sliced red onion.

Serves 4 to 6

Boldly Brilliant Borscht
. . . .

INGREDIENTS:

1 large beet, peeled and chopped

1 medium tomato, chopped

1 small apple (such as Ida Red or Empire), peeled, cored, and
chopped

1 large stalk celery, chopped

1 (1-inch) knob ginger, chopped

1 or 2 small cloves garlic, chopped

½ teaspoon salt (or to taste)

¼ teaspoon ground coriander

2 tablespoons freshly squeezed lemon juice, or 1 tablespoon
raw unfiltered apple cider vinegar

1 cup water

1 large carrot, grated

½ cup grated or shredded cabbage (red or green or mix of both)

OPTIONAL:

¼ to ½ teaspoon (or more) cracked black pepper or cayenne
pepper

½ cup or more sauerkraut (if using this, eliminate salt)

½ cup Caesar Cashew Ranch Dressing (page 244)

1 ripe medium avocado, sliced or cubed

GARNISH:

2 tablespoons finely chopped fresh dill

LOVING PREPARATION:

1. Put the beet, tomato, apple, celery, ginger, garlic, salt, coriander,
lemon juice, and pepper (if using) in a blender and blend. As the
mixture is blending, gently pour the water through the top opening. Blend until completely liquefied.
2. Transfer to a large bowl and stir in the carrot and cabbage and/
or optional sauerkraut.

3. To serve, pour into individual bowls and add a dollop of cashew dressing or a few slices of avocado, if desired. Garnish with dill and serve. Borscht can be refrigerated for up to 5 days. In fact, this soup often tastes better the next day when flavors have had a chance to meld.

NOTE Most of the time, a standard blender works just fine in a Good Karma kitchen. This is one dish in which you will notice a more perfect texture if you have a high-powered blender.

Makes 5 cups

Sensational Salads and Dazzling Dressings

When people mention being vegan, and certainly when the topic of raw food comes up, someone is likely to say, "Oh, you must eat a lot of salad," with a subtext of, "I'm glad I don't have to eat all that salad." But this is because there's salad—and then there's *salad*—glorious greenery with so many additions and nuances, you really do want to eat it first.

Caesar Salad with Cashew Ranch
. . . .

DRESSING INGREDIENTS:

1 cup raw cashews, soaked for 4 hours, rinsed, and drained
2 tablespoons raw unfiltered apple cider vinegar
2 tablespoons freshly squeezed lemon juice

¾ cup water (for a dressing consistency)

¼ teaspoon cracked black pepper

2 pitted dates, soaked for 10 minutes, or 1 teaspoon maple
syrup

1 or 2 cloves garlic, chopped

½ teaspoon dry dill weed

1 teaspoon dulse or kelp flakes

SALAD INGREDIENTS:

4 cups chopped romaine lettuce

8 cherry tomatoes, halved

¼ cup ground pumpkin seeds

¼ cup slivered almonds, raw or toasted

LOVING PREPARATION:

1. For the dressing: Put all the ingredients except the dry dill weed and dulse in a blender and blend until smooth and creamy. If using a regular blender (not a high-powered one, such as a Vita-mix), add the water gradually through the opening at the top, to prevent it from splashing out and overflowing.
2. Add the dry dill and dulse, and blend briefly to combine.
3. For the salad: Toss the lettuce with a portion of the dressing, enough to coat the leaves but leaving some dressing to top the salads. Place the dressed lettuce and tomato halves in individual bowls and drizzle 2 to 3 tablespoons of the remaining dressing on top of each. Sprinkle on top 1 to 2 teaspoons per serving of ground pumpkin seeds (to mimic Parmesan) and 1 tablespoon slivered almonds (for a crouton-like crunch).

VARIATION

This dressing recipe also makes a perfect ranch dip—just decrease the amount of water you use from ¾ cup to ⅓ cup.

Makes 2 large or 4 small servings

Kale-idoscope Salad
· · · · · · · ·

DRESSING INGREDIENTS:

3 tablespoons olive oil, plus more if needed

1 medium avocado

¼ cup freshly squeezed lemon juice, plus more if needed

1 tablespoon organic or non-GMO tamari

1 tablespoon grated fresh ginger, or ½ teaspoon ginger powder

1 clove garlic, minced (optional)

SALAD INGREDIENTS:

4 cups tightly packed chopped kale

½ cup steamed and chopped cauliflower

1 small carrot, grated

2 cups sliced radishes

2 tablespoons finely chopped fresh parsley

Salt and freshly ground black pepper

2 tablespoons hempseeds

2 tablespoons pumpkin seeds

LOVING PREPARATION:

1. For the dressing: In a small bowl, mix the olive oil, avocado, lemon juice, tamari, ginger, and garlic (if using) until creamy. (Lemon juice helps break down the tough fibers in cruciferous greens such as kale, making them easier to chew and digest.)
2. For the salad: In a large bowl, massage the kale with the dressing until it begins to wilt. If it's too dry, add a little more lemon juice and olive oil.
3. Add the cauliflower, carrot, radishes, and parsley and toss together well. Sprinkle with salt and pepper to your preference, then serve on a plate.
4. Sprinkle with hemp and pumpkin seeds.

Serves 2 to 4

One Wondrous Waldorf

·········

DRESSING INGREDIENTS:

1 medium avocado, mashed

2 tablespoon freshly squeezed lemon juice

1 teaspoon Dijon mustard, or ½ teaspoon dry mustard

1 teaspoon chopped fresh parsley

½ to 1 teaspoon white horseradish (optional, for a bit of kick—see note)

1 tablespoon olive oil

SALAD INGREDIENTS:

2 medium red or green apples, diced

1 large stalk celery, diced small or thinly sliced

1 cup seedless grapes (red or green—try a contrasting color to apples), halved

½ cup walnuts or cashews, raw or toasted, coarsely chopped

3 cups chopped or torn romaine lettuce

1 head Belgian endive, leaves separated

2 tablespoons hempseeds (optional)

LOVING PREPARATION:

1. For the dressing: In a medium bowl, mash together the avocado, 1 tablespoon of the lemon juice, the mustard, parsley, and horse-radish (if using).

2. Mix together the olive oil with the remaining 1 tablespoon lemon juice and set aside.

3. For the salad: In a medium bowl, combine the apples, celery, grapes, and nuts.

4. Add the dressing to the salad and mix until the apples and greens are evenly coated.

5. To serve, place the lettuce on a serving platter or individual plates, and arrange the endive leaves in a wheel on top of the romaine. Place the apple mixture in the center of the platter and top with a few more walnuts and a sprinkle of hempseeds (if using).

NOTE Horseradish: Grate fresh horseradish or buy it bottled at a European deli or the kosher section of a supermarket.

Serves 3 to 4

Cheesy Caprese

·········

INGREDIENTS:

1 (1-pound) block non-GMO extra-firm tofu, drained

2 tablespoons organic balsamic or red wine vinegar

1 teaspoon salt, plus more for serving

4 medium vine ripe or Roma tomatoes, cut into ¼-inch-thick circles

⅓ cup fresh basil leaves, chopped, plus 4 to 6 additional whole leaves for decoration

Olive oil, for drizzling

Cracked black pepper (optional)

½ lemon

LOVING PREPARATION:

1. Halve the tofu block lengthwise, then cut each half into 12 equal slices.

2. In a shallow bowl, stir the vinegar with the salt until the salt has completely dissolved. Dip each slice of tofu into the vinegar and transfer the slices to a rack set over a rimmed baking sheet. Refrigerate, uncovered, for 8 hours or overnight to dry to a more mozzarella-like consistency and to absorb the seasonings.

3. Fan out the tomatoes on a large platter in a circle or a long row, overlapping one another. Tuck the tofu slices between the tomato slices and sprinkle the chopped basil leaves on top. Drizzle your salad with olive oil and sprinkle with salt and pepper, if you'd like. Squeeze a bit of fresh lemon juice on top, garnish with the whole basil leaves, and serve.

NOTE Add a few dollops of Presto Pesto (page 254) to complement and enhance the flavor even more.

VARIATION

Instead of tofu, slice 2 ripe medium avocados into about 24 slices and skip the marinating process and lemon juice. Tuck the avocado between the tomato slices, drizzle with vinegar and olive oil, sprinkle with salt and pepper, and enjoy.

Serves 4 to 6

Three-Bean Supreme
. . . .

SALAD INGREDIENTS:

½ cup each cooked black beans, black-eyed peas, chickpeas, or other beans (see note)
¼ cup diced red onion
¼ cup scallion, finely sliced
1 stalk celery, diced
1 medium carrot, grated
3 radishes, sliced
2 tablespoons finely chopped fresh parsley
2 tablespoons finely chopped fresh cilantro

DRESSING INGREDIENTS:

2 tablespoons olive oil
2 tablespoons tahini
¼ cup freshly squeezed orange juice

2 teaspoons apple cider vinegar, or 2 tablespoons freshly
squeezed lemon juice

1 tablespoon organic mild miso or tamari

Salt and freshly ground black pepper

OPTIONAL:

½ teaspoon dried rosemary

1 clove garlic, minced

LOVING PREPARATION:

1. For the salad: Combine all the salad ingredients in a large bowl.
2. For the dressing: Put the dressing ingredients except the salt and pepper in a jar with a secure lid, cover, and shake to combine; add the rosemary and/or garlic (if using) and shake once more to combine. Mix the dressing gently into the bean salad. Taste and add salt and pepper as you like.
3. Let stand at room temperature for 20 minutes before serving, to absorb the dressing and allow the flavor to deepen. This salad often tastes better the next day, and it will keep in your fridge for up to 3 days.

NOTE Ideal method for cooking dry beans: Lentils, split peas, and split mung dahl can be cooked without soaking first. For other beans, soak overnight in 3 times more water than beans. Rinse and strain, then boil in 2 times more water than beans for 4 minutes. Remove from the heat and keep the pot covered for 3 to 4 hours. Rinse and strain, then add enough water to cover the beans by ½ inch. Bring to a boil; reduce the heat to medium and cook for 30 minutes to 1 hour (depending on the type of bean). This method is prized by natural-food cooks as the way to cut down on beans' tendency to cause gassiness. Adding a piece of seaweed or kombu or a bit of the herb savory may help with this as well. And you can save time by making a large batch and freezing the cooked beans to quickly reheat later. (A pressure cooker will cut cooking time in half. If you have one, or if you're thinking of getting one, check out *The New Fast Food*, by Jill Nussinow, MS, RD, and *Vegan Pressure Cooking*, by JL Fields.)

Serves 4 to 6

Dips, Spreads, and Pâtés

Raw dips and pâtés are scrumptious—and so easy. Scoop on top of a salad or serve with raw veggies; use for sandwiches and wraps, or as a stuffing for tomatoes, peppers, or mushrooms.

Save-the-Tuna Salad
....

INGREDIENTS:

   1½ cups sunflower seeds, soaked for 4 hours, rinsed and
      drained
   3 tablespoons freshly squeezed lemon juice
   2 cloves garlic, minced
   2 teaspoons dulse flakes or granules
   ¼ teaspoon cracked black pepper
   ¼ cup red onion, chopped
   1 stalk celery, diced
   A handful of your favorite fresh herbs (dill, parsley, cilantro,
      etc.), finely chopped (optional)

Salt (if needed—dulse flakes impart a salty flavor)

Whole-grain bread, leaf wrap (Swiss chard, collard, romaine lettuce, or cabbage leaf), crudités, or crackers, for serving

LOVING PREPARATION:

1. Combine the seeds, lemon juice, garlic, dulse, and pepper in a food processor and process until smooth. (Process less if you like it chunky.)
2. Transfer the mixture to a medium bowl and stir in the onion, celery, and fresh herbs (if using). Taste, and add more salt if necessary.
3. Spread on whole-grain bread for a sandwich, or into a leaf wrap; it may also be served with crudités or crackers. The spread will keep in the refrigerator for up to 1 week.

Makes 2 cups

Top-Drawer Tapenade
·········

INGREDIENTS:

1 cup pitted Kalamata or black olives (canned, jarred, fresh, cured, or mixed), rinsed and drained (see notes)

2 tablespoons capers, rinsed well and drained (see notes)

2 teaspoons freshly squeezed lemon juice

1 or 2 cloves garlic, minced

2 tablespoons chopped fresh parsley, or 5 fresh basil leaves

2 tablespoons olive oil (or the oil from oil-packed olives)

Salt (optional)

LOVING PREPARATION:

1. In a food processor, blend all the ingredients except the salt. Scrape down the sides of the bowl as necessary. Don't allow the texture to become creamy: traditional tapenade is a little chunky. Taste the mixture first before adding additional salt. The saltiness of the olives is often enough.

NOTES Olives: Read the can or package ingredients carefully. Olives are usually sold in a brine of salt, water, and vinegar (often red wine vinegar) and sometimes olive oil. Salt is a natural preservative, so try to avoid the ones with added preservatives. The organic olives you can buy at health food stores are usually excellent; so are many of the varieties found in European delis, or sold scoop-and-weigh style at olive bars in select grocery stores. If using cured (or dried) olives, soak in water for 15 minutes to remove some of the excess salt. Then drain and gently pat dry.

   Capers: As with olives, avoid those with artificial preservatives. Capers are routinely oversalted for preservation purposes, so soak them in water for 15 minutes to remove excess salt, drain, and gently pat dry before using.

Makes 1 cup

Presto Pesto

· · · · · · · ·

INGREDIENTS:

   2 cups tightly packed fresh basil leaves, rinsed and dried (see note)

1½ cups tightly packed kale leaves (flat or curly) or baby
   spinach, rinsed and dried

¼ cup freshly squeezed lemon juice

⅓ cup olive oil

1 to 2 cloves garlic, chopped

1 cup raw walnuts, soaked for 4 hours, rinsed, drained, and
   dried

1 teaspoon salt (or to taste)

LOVING PREPARATION:

1. In a food processor, process all the ingredients until smooth and
   creamy, or process less for a chunky texture. Scrape down the
   sides of the bowl as necessary. Stored in a glass jar in the fridge,
   this pesto keeps for up to 2 weeks. Or freeze in an airtight plastic
   container, with a thin layer of olive oil poured on top to prevent
   freezer burn.

NOTE Presto Pesto is delicious with any savory food: add to salad
dressings, sauces, soups, spreads, dips, pâtés, pasta, sautéed veggies, scrambled tofu—even toast!

Makes 2 cups

Marvelous Mains

These heavier dishes can center your meal quite nicely, and having a
repertoire of them is especially important when you're new to meatless dining.

Potatoful

....

INGREDIENTS:

4 medium sweet potatoes or yams, whole and unpeeled

1 medium red onion, peeled and diced

2 tablespoons olive oil

1 cup non-GMO soft tofu, paper towel dried and cubed

1 small red bell pepper, diced small

1 cup broccoli florets, chopped small

1 stalk celery, diced small

¼ cup freshly squeezed orange juice

1 tablespoon grated fresh ginger, or ½ teaspoon powdered
   ginger

1 tablespoon tahini

1 tablespoon non-GMO miso, or 1 teaspoon salt

GARNISHES:

Sweet Hungarian paprika

Fresh or dried parsley

"Rawmesan" or "Parma!"—commercially available vegan
   Parmesans

LOVING PREPARATION:

1. Steam the potatoes whole and unpeeled for 25 minutes. Allow
   them to cool completely.
2. Meanwhile, sauté the onion in the olive oil over medium heat
   until golden brown.
3. Add the tofu and sauté for 10 minutes more.

4. Reduce the temperature and add the bell peppers, broccoli, and celery. Sauté, stirring occasionally, for 5 minutes more.

5. Combine the orange juice, ginger, tahini, and miso in a bowl, then add to the tofu/vegetable mixture. Stir well and keep covered.

6. Halve the potatoes vertically down the middle, but not all the way through—you're making a "bed" or a "boat" to hold the prepared veggies. Scoop out about half the flesh from each side of the potatoes and mix it with the tofu/vegetable stuffing.

7. Fill the potatoes with the stuffing, and top with one or more of the suggested garnishes.

Serves 4 as an entrée. If you cut all the way through the potatoes and stuff the halves, this becomes a side dish serving 8.

Curried Buckwheat Pilaf
. . . .

INGREDIENTS:

3 tablespoons olive oil

1 tablespoon whole mustard seeds (black or yellow)

2 tablespoons unsalted curry powder (see note)

½ teaspoon ground cinnamon

1 teaspoon ground cumin

¼ cup water

3 medium shallots, sliced

2½ cups boiling water

1 to 2 teaspoons salt (or to taste)

1 cup buckwheat, rinsed (or use quinoa:
   see Variation)

2 cups chopped vegetables (asparagus, broccoli, Brussels sprouts, snow peas, carrots, celery, green beans, etc.)

⅓ cup chopped fresh cilantro

LOVING PREPARATION:

1. In a medium pot, heat the oil over medium-low heat. Add the seeds, curry powder, cinnamon, and cumin and cook, stirring continuously, for 3 to 4 minutes, being careful that they do not burn. If the oil smokes, the heat is too high.
2. Add the ¼ cup water and shallots. Bring to a boil, stir, keep covered, reduce the temperature, and cook, stirring occasionally, for 5 minutes.
3. Increase the temperature to medium and add the 2½ cups boiling water, plus the salt and buckwheat. Stir, bring to a boil, cover, reduce the temperature to medium-low, and simmer for 10 minutes.
4. Remove from the heat and keep covered for 10 minutes more. In the meantime, prepare the vegetables (rinse, peel, chop) and add them to the pot. Mix well, but gently.
5. Reduce the heat to low, cover, and cook, stirring occasionally, for 5 minutes.
6. Remove from the heat. Add the cilantro and stir. Let stand, covered, for 5 minutes more. Enjoy!

VARIATION

For a Curried Quinoa Pilaf, replace the buckwheat with 1 cup rinsed quinoa and add 2 cups boiling water instead of 2½ cups.

NOTE There are many different kinds of curry powders: Jamaican, Indian, Sri Lankan, Nepalese, Thai, etc. Try different kinds of curries, opt for organic where possible, and avoid those with added preservatives, salt, or MSG.

If you want to make your own curry powder, the primary ingredients of a standard curry are cumin and coriander, with turmeric to taste (this antioxidant and anti-inflammatory spice gives curry its characteristic yellow hue) and a touch of dry mustard, powdered ginger, and cayenne or crushed red pepper flakes.

Serves 4 to 6

Thai Greens and Beans
·········

INGREDIENTS:

1 medium red onion, thinly sliced

½ cup water, or 1½ tablespoons olive oil, for sautéing

1 cup each shiitake and oyster mushrooms, sliced (or use any combo of mushrooms)

Vegetable broth, cooking wine, or water, as needed

1 cup broccoli florets

1 stalk celery, chopped

1 cup baby bok choy, leaves separated (approximately 2 heads)

1 can garbanzo beans (chickpeas)

2 teaspoons quality toasted sesame seed oil (see note)

1 tablespoon tahini (sesame paste)

1 tablespoon tamari or shoyu (natural soy sauce)

2 tablespoons freshly squeezed lemon juice

2 or 3 small cloves garlic, minced

½ teaspoon ginger powder

1 tablespoon sesame seeds, toasted

LOVING PREPARATION:

1. Sauté the onion in olive oil, or steam-sauté it in water, in a large covered skillet over medium-low heat for 5 minutes. Add the mushrooms. Stir and continue to sauté for 10 minutes more, adding the vegetable broth to provide enough liquid to keep the onions and mushrooms from sticking or burning.
2. Add, in this order, the broccoli, celery, and bok choy. Reduce the temperature slightly. *Do not stir.* Cover and cook for 5 minutes. (The temperature should be low to prevent scorching or overcooking the veggies.)
3. Drain the garbanzo beans (chickpeas) and stir them into the vegetables, adding a bit of broth if necessary to keep from sticking,
4. Meanwhile, mix the sesame oil, tahini, tamari, lemon juice, garlic, and ginger in a bowl. Remove from the heat, add the sauce, and mix well to cover the greens evenly. Cover for 2 minutes and serve with a sprinkle of toasted sesame seeds.

NOTE Do not use sesame seed oil, or any oil, for that matter, that has been open for longer than 3 months. Oils go rancid very easily due to oxidization, especially when toasted. Keep your sesame oil refrigerated after opening and away from direct sunlight. Buy in a glass bottle only, preferably a dark glass bottle.

Serves 2 generously

Firehouse Stew

. . . .

2 tablespoons olive oil

½ cup red onions, thinly sliced

1 teaspoon finely diced jalapeño pepper (more or less
   depending on your taste and heat tolerance)

2 medium tomatoes, diced

½ cup water

2 cups extra-firm tofu, drained, patted dry, and cubed

2 stalks celery, sliced on an angle

½ cup carrots, sliced on an angle

½ cup peas

½ cup diced zucchini

2 or 3 cloves garlic, minced

1½ teaspoons salt

2 tablespoons chopped fresh cilantro, plus more for garnish

LOVING PREPARATION:

1. Heat the olive oil in a skillet over medium-low heat, and sauté the
   onions and jalapeño, stirring occasionally, for 10 minutes.
2. Add the tomatoes. Stir and cover; continue to cook, stirring
   occasionally, for 10 minutes more. Add the water, stir, and bring
   to a boil.
3. Add the tofu, cover, and cook for 5 minutes more.
4. Reduce the heat to maintain a simmer and add the celery, carrots, peas, and zucchini. Cover and continue to simmer for 2
   minutes.
5. Add the garlic and salt and stir. Remove from the heat, cover,
   and let stand for 5 minutes.

6. Add the cilantro and stir.
7. Serve on a bed of quinoa, amaranth, buckwheat, or brown rice and garnish with fresh cilantro.

NOTE If you love cilantro, you love it a lot. Some 10 percent of folks, however, lack an enzyme required for enjoying this green herb. To them, it tastes like soap. When preparing a dish that calls for cilantro for company, you may opt to leave it out or substitute curly parsley or perhaps arugula.

Serves 4

Veggie Sidekicks

In vegetarian cuisine, the lines can blur about just what role a particular dish plays in a meal. You may want to make a big batch of one of these side dishes to serve as a main course, or to top a bowl of fresh greens, thereby creating a "whole-meal salad." If you desire a source of concentrated protein in an all-vegetable meal, toss some beans or seared tofu into your salad; add some veggie-meat to a side vegetable; have baked beans or black beans as a side dish; or start lunch or dinner with lentil soup.

Broccoli Italiano
· · · · · · · ·

INGREDIENTS:

5 cups broccoli florets
½ teaspoon dried rosemary
¼ teaspoon dried thyme

¼ teaspoon dried oregano

1 tablespoon olive oil

1 tablespoon freshly squeezed lemon juice

1 tablespoon toasted sesame seeds (optional)

1. Steam the florets for 3 to 4 minutes over gently boiling water. Remove right away and rinse with cold water (to prevent the broccoli from cooking further), then drain. If you prefer warm, steam for 2 minutes and skip the rinse procedure.

2. Stir together the rosemary, thyme, oregano, olive oil, and lemon juice in a bowl.

3. Transfer the broccoli to a medium bowl and pour the herb mixture over the top. Mix and massage gently and thoroughly with your hands or with two spoons.

4. Sprinkle with sesame seeds, if you'd like, then serve immediately.

Smashed Potatoes

. . . .

INGREDIENTS:

6 medium yellow Finn potatoes, unpeeled

¼ cup unsweetened almond milk (or other unsweetened vegan milk)

½ teaspoon salt (or to taste)

1 or 2 small cloves garlic, minced

¼ to ½ teaspoon cracked black pepper or cayenne pepper (optional)

2 tablespoons finely chopped fresh dill or parsley, to garnish

1. Place the potatoes in a steaming rack over gently boiling water; the water should not touch the potatoes. Reduce the heat just enough to keep a gentle boil going. Steam, covered, for 20 to 25 minutes, or until the potatoes are tender. Pierce the thickest part in the center of a potato to check its tenderness. It shouldn't be too soft (overdone) or too hard (underdone).
2. Remove the potatoes from the pot and cover them with a towel for 5 minutes, to remove excess steam and prevent sogginess. Allow to cool slightly, then peel and coarsely chop.
3. In a bowl, whip together the potatoes, almond milk, salt, garlic, and pepper (if using) either by hand with a potato masher or with an electric mixer, to the desired consistency.
4. Garnish each portion with fresh dill before serving.

VARIATION

Instead of 4 potatoes, whip 3; then add the flesh from a ripe medium avocado and whip again, just until combined. This way, you'll get your healthy fats and extra creaminess—delightful!

Makes about 4 cups; serves 4 to 6

Candied Carrots
········

INGREDIENTS:

1 tablespoon olive oil
1 medium red onion, peeled and thinly sliced

2 medium carrots, peeled and cut into coins (approximately
   2 cups)

¼ cup water

3 tablespoons maple syrup

1 teaspoon ground cinnamon

¼ teaspoon vanilla bean powder, or 1 teaspoon vanilla extract

LOVING PREPARATION:

1. Heat the olive oil in a skillet over medium-low heat. Add the onion
   and sauté, stirring occasionally, until golden brown, 10 to 12
   minutes.
2. Add the carrots, water, and 2 tablespoons of the maple syrup.
   Stir, cover, and cook for 10 minutes.
3. Add the remaining 1 tablespoon maple syrup, the cinnamon,
   and the vanilla. Stir. Remove from the heat, cover, and let stand
   for 5 minutes before serving. May be served hot or cold.

Serves 2 to 4

Masquerading Mashed "Potatoes"
. . . .

INGREDIENTS:

4 cups chopped cauliflower florets

½ cup raw cashews, soaked for 4 hours, rinsed, and drained

2 small cloves garlic, chopped (if you like it garlicky, add more)

½ teaspoon salt (add more to your taste)

¼ teaspoon cracked black pepper, plus more for serving

½ teaspoon dried rosemary

2 tablespoons olive oil

2 teaspoons raw unfiltered apple cider vinegar

2 tablespoons finely chopped fresh dill, or 1 teaspoon dried dill
(optional), plus a sprig of fresh dill or parsley for garnish

LOVING PREPARATION:

1. Combine all the ingredients except the dill (if using) in a food processor and process until smooth and creamy. Scrape down the
sides of the bowl as necessary. Taste, adding more salt if desired.
Transfer to a bowl and mix in the dill (if using).

2. Serve with a sprinkle of black pepper and a garnish of dill or
parsley.

Serves 4

Desserts to Live For

Raw desserts are, simply, heaven on earth. They're full of real-food
ingredients and since they're usually based on fruit, with its own
delightful sweetness, they depend less on concentrated sweeteners of
any sort. They're also incredibly easy to make. Gone are the days of
the cake that didn't rise or the piecrust that didn't hold together: these
recipes will work every time and win over any skeptic.

Banana Soft Serve

....

INGREDIENTS:

4 ripe bananas, frozen

1 teaspoon vanilla extract, or ¼ teaspoon vanilla bean powder

4 tablespoons nut milk (almond/Brazil) or water

OPTIONAL:

For a chocolate version: 1 tablespoon raw fair-trade cacao powder

GARNISH:

1 tablespoon unsulfured, unsweetened, dried coconut shreds

1 tablespoon chopped nuts (almonds, walnuts, hazelnuts, etc.)

Cacao powder

LOVING PREPARATION:

1. Combine the bananas, vanilla, nut milk, and cacao (if using) in a food processor or powerful blender with a tamper, and process until smooth and creamy like ice cream. Scrape down the sides of the bowl so that all the banana is puréed.

2. When the mixture reaches the consistency of soft-serve ice cream, scoop it into serving dishes and sprinkle, if you like, with coconut, nuts, or a bit more cacao powder.

Make a sundae with the addition of a drizzle of maple syrup or chocolate syrup (Cè Organics makes a delicious one with fair-trade ingredients).

Drizzle with a nice brandy for a sophisticated grown-up dessert.

Serves 2 to 4

Tropical Ambrosia
....

INGREDIENTS:

1 ripe medium mango, peeled, pit removed, and flesh
   chopped into chunks
1 medium grapefruit or orange, peeled and chopped
½ cup pineapple chunks
½ cup berries (strawberries, blueberries, or any other you like)
1 cup melon seeds (see notes)
½ teaspoon ground cinnamon
¼ teaspoon vanilla bean powder, or 1 teaspoon vanilla extract
1 tablespoon freshly squeezed lemon juice
¼ cup chopped almonds or other nut
1 tablespoon finely chopped fresh mint leaves

OPTIONAL:

1 tablespoon maple syrup or 4 pitted dates, soaked for 10
   minutes and drained
1 (1-inch) piece fresh ginger, chopped

LOVING PREPARATION:

1. In a large bowl, toss together the mango, grapefruit, pineapple, berries, and/or any other fruit you like (see notes).
2. Make the cream by blending the melon seeds, cinnamon, vanilla, lemon juice, and any of the optional ingredients until smooth and creamy. Taste and adjust the seasonings if necessary.
3. Pour the cream into the fruit and stir until evenly coated.
4. To serve, spoon the mixture into individual bowls and sprinkle with nuts and chopped fresh mint. If you're serving company, add a mint leaf for decoration and a teeny drizzle of maple syrup.

VARIATION

If you want to skip the melon seeds, obtain the creamy texture by using an additional ½ cup chopped mango or ½ cup chopped pineapple instead.

NOTES Fruits: Try any combination of tropical fruits or, if you prefer to eat locally, make this with seasonal fruits native to your region: peaches, plums, apples, pears, berries, melon, etc.

Melon seeds: Filled with vitamins, minerals, protein, and fiber, these make a fabulous cream. There are many melons to choose from. Some of my favorites are the seeds from cantaloupe, honeydew, and yellow canary melons. These seeds are also delicious dried and lightly toasted.

Almonds, or any other nut you like, can be used in ambrosia. Ideally, the nuts will be soaked overnight, rinsed, and drained before using. If you like the toasted flavor, lightly toast dry, chopped nuts in a dry skillet over medium-low heat until lightly browned and fragrant.

Serves 3 or 4

Pie in the Sky

· · · · · · · ·

CRUST INGREDIENTS:

- 1 cup pitted dates (if too dry, soak in warm water for 20 minutes and drain)
- 1 cup raw hazelnuts, pecans, or walnuts, soaked for 4 to 6 hours, rinsed, and drained

FILLING INGREDIENTS:

- 2 ripe medium avocados
- 2 teaspoons vanilla extract, or ½ teaspoon vanilla bean
- ⅔ cup freshly squeezed lemon juice
- 1 teaspoon freshly grated lemon zest
- ⅓ cup maple syrup, or ½ cup pitted dates
- 1 cup raw cashews, soaked for 4 hours, rinsed, and drained

TOPPINGS:

- 1 cup berries (raspberries, blueberries, blackberries, strawberries, etc.)
- 2 cups seasonal fruit slices (apples, peaches, pears, plums, cherries, etc.)

LOVING PREPARATION:

1. For the crust: Combine the dates and nuts in a food processor and process until a ball forms. The nuts should be chunky.

2. Cover a 7- or 8-inch pie dish with plastic wrap and press the date-nut mixture evenly into the pan. Refrigerate while preparing the filling.
3. For the filling: Puree the avocados, vanilla, lemon juice, lemon zest, and sweetener in a food processor until creamy. Add the cashews and continue to blend until creamy.
4. Pour or scoop the filling mixture into the prepared crust. Wiggle and whack the dish on the countertop to spread the filling evenly.
5. Freeze for 4 hours or overnight. Remove the plastic wrap and place on a serving dish before decorating.
6. Before serving, decorate with toppings, piling the fruit high.
7. This delicacy thaws quickly, so it can be served frozen, half frozen, or completely thawed as a custard pie.

Makes one 7- or 8-inch pie

Peaches and Cream
. . . .

INGREDIENTS:

1 cup raw cashews or cashew pieces, soaked for 4 hours, rinsed, and drained
3 tablespoons maple syrup
3 tablespoons freshly squeezed lemon juice
¼ teaspoon ground cardamom
1 teaspoon vanilla extract, or ¼ teaspoon vanilla bean
6 medium peaches, pitted, peeled, and sliced

LOVING PREPARATION:

1. Combine the cashews, maple syrup, lemon juice, cardamom, and vanilla in a food processor and process until smooth and creamy.
2. To serve, spoon the peaches evenly into individual bowls and top each with 2 tablespoons of the cream. A nice garnish might be a sprinkle of cardamom and a mint leaf. You can refrigerate the cream in an airtight container for up to 1 week—if there are any leftovers.

Serves 4 to 6

Chocolate Bliss Balls

· · · · · · · ·

INGREDIENTS:

    1 cup almonds, walnuts, or other raw nuts, soaked for 4 to 6
        hours, rinsed, drained, and dried
    1 cup dates, pitted and chopped (if too dry, soak for 30
        minutes and drain before chopping)
    ½ cup cocoa powder (ideally raw, fair-trade cacao), plus more
        for rolling

OPTIONAL:

    ½ cup dried, unsulfured, shredded coconut, plus more for
        rolling
    1 teaspoon ground cinnamon
    1 teaspoon freshly grated lemon or orange zest (use organic)
    ¼ teaspoon freshly grated nutmeg

½ teaspoon ginger powder

½ cup ground nuts, for rolling

LOVING PREPARATION:

1. Pulse the nuts in a food processor until roughly chopped. Add the dates, cocoa powder, and any optional ingredients and process until a ball forms.
2. Roll the mixture into balls of your desired size, then roll the balls in cacao powder, shredded coconut, or ground nuts. Store in an airtight container in the refrigerator for up to 1 week.

VARIATION

To make protein balls or bars, add a few scoops of vegan protein powder during the blending.

Makes 15 to 25 bliss balls

Appendix B

......

Books for Your Bedside and for Your Kitchen

Recommended Reading

Note: I've attempted to separate the books from the cookbooks, but many of the "Recommended Reading" selections have great recipes, and the "Recommended Eating" offerings contain a plethora of wisdom along with the recipes.

Adams, Carol J., Patti Breitman, and Virginia Messina, MPH, RD. *Never Too Late to Go Vegan: The Over-50 Guide to Adopting and Thriving on a Plant-Based Diet.* New York: The Experiment, 2014.

Baur, Gene, and Gene Stone. *Living the Farm Sanctuary Life: The Ultimate Guide to Eating Mindfully, Living Longer, and Feeling Better Every Day.* New York: Rodale, 2015.

Bisci, Fred, PhD. *Your Health Journey: Discovering Your Body's Full Potential.* New York: Bisci Lifestyle Books, 2009.

Campbell, T. Colin, PhD, with Howard Jacobson, PhD. *The Low-Carb Fraud.* Dallas: BenBella Books, 2014.

———. *Whole: Rethinking the Science of Nutrition.* Dallas: BenBella Books, 2014.

Cheeke, Robert. *Shred It! Burning Fat and Building Muscle on a Plant-Based Diet.* Los Angeles: Gaven Press, 2014.

Colb, Sherry, JD. *Mind If I Order the Cheeseburger?* New York: Lantern Books, 2013.

Cooney, Nick. *Veganomics: The Surprising Science Behind What Motivates Vegetarians, from the Breakfast Table to the Bedroom.* New York: Lantern Books, 2013.

Davis, Brenda, RD, and Vesanto Melina, MS, RD, with Rynn Berry. *Becoming Raw: The Essential Guide to Raw Vegan Diets.* Summertown, TN: Book Publishing Company, 2010.

———. *Becoming Vegan: Express Edition, The Everyday Guide to Plant-Based Nutrition.* Summertown, TN: Book Publishing Company, 2013.

Dinshah, H. Jay, and Anne Dinshah. *Powerful Vegan Messages.* Malaga, NJ: American Vegan Society, 2014.

Ferrante, Frank. *May I Be Frank: How I Changed My Ways, Lost 100 Pounds, and Found Love Again.* Berkeley, CA: North Atlantic Books, 2015.

Freston, Kathy. *The Lean: A Revolutionary (and Simple!) 30-Day Plan for Healthy, Lasting Weight Loss.* New York: Weinstein Books, 2012.

Fuhrman, Joel, MD. *The End of Dieting: How to Live for Life.* San Francisco: HarperOne, 2014.

Fuhrman, Talia. *Love Your Body: Eat Smart, Get Healthy, Find Your Ideal Weight, and Feel Beautiful Inside & Out.* New York: Rodale, 2014.

Golfman, Jeff. *The Cool Vegetarian: The Ultimate Guide for a Veggie, Vegan & Raw Life.* Toronto: Jeff Golfman, 2013.

Gruno, Brad. *Brad's Raw Made Easy: The Fast, Delicious Way to Lose Weight, Optimize Health, and Live Mostly in the Raw.* New York: Harmony Books, 2014.

Hever, Julieanna, MS, RD. *The Vegiterranean Diet: The New and Improved Mediterranean Eating Plan—with Deliciously Satisfying Vegan Recipes for Optimal Health.* Boston: DaCapo Lifelong, 2014.

Hicks, J. Morris. *Healthy Eating, Healthy World: Unleashing the Power of Plant-Based Nutrition.* Dallas: BenBella Books, 2011.

Joseph, John. *Meat Is for Pussies: A How-to Guide for Dudes Who Want to Get Fit, Kick Ass, and Take Names.* New York: HarperWave, 2014.

Kahn, Joel, MD. *The Whole Heart Solution: A Preventive Cardiologist's Guide to Halt Heart Disease Now.* New York: Reader's Digest Books, 2014.

Kanner, Ellen. *Feeding the Hungry Ghost: Life, Faith, and What to Eat for Dinner.* Novato, CA: New World Library, 2013.

Messina, Virginia, MPH, RD, with JL Fields, VLCE. *Vegan for Her: The Woman's Guide to Being Healthy and Fit on a Plant-Based Diet.* Boston: DaCapo Lifelong, 2013.

Moran, Victoria. *The Love-Powered Diet: Eating for Freedom, Health, and Joy.* New York: Lantern Books, 2009.

———. *Main Street Vegan: Everything You Need to Know to Eat Healthfully and Live Compassionately in the Real World.* New York: Tarcher/Penguin, 2012.

Norris, Jack, RD, and Virginia Messina, MPH, RD. *Vegan for Life: Everything You Need to Know to Be Healthy and Fit on a Plant-Based Diet.* Boston: DaCapo Lifelong, 2011.

Oppenlander, Richard A., DDS. *Comfortably Unaware: What We Eat Is Killing Us and Our Planet.* New York: Beaufort Books, 2012.

Patrick-Goudreau, Colleen. *The 30-Day Vegan Challenge: The Ultimate Guide to Eating Healthfully and Living Compassionately.* Oakland, CA: Montali Press, 2014.

Pierre, John. *The Pillars of Health: Your Foundations for Lifelong Wellness.* Carlsbad, CA, and New York: Hay House, 2013.

Popper, Pamela, PhD, ND, and Glen Merzer. *Food over Medicine: The Conversation That Could Save Your Life.* Dallas: BenBella Books, 2014.

Quivers, Robin. *The Vegucation of Robin: How Real Food Saved My Life.* New York: Avery, 2013.

Rose, Natalia. *Forever Beautiful: The Age-Defying Detox Plan.* Guilford, CT: Skirt! 2014.

Simon, David Robinson. *Meatonomics: How the Rigged Economics of Meat and Dairy Make You Consume Too Much—and How to Eat Better, Live Longer, and Spend Smarter.* Berkeley, CA: Conari Press, 2013.

Tuttle, Will, PhD, ed. *Circles of Compassion: Connecting Issues of Justice.* Boston: Vegan Publishers, 2014.

Uliano, Sophie. *Gorgeous for Good: A Simple 30-Day Program for Lasting Beauty Inside and Out.* Carlsbad, CA: Hay House, 2015.

Wolfe, David. *Eating for Beauty.* Berkeley, CA: North Atlantic Books, 2009.

Recommend Eating

Asbell, Robin. *Juice It! Energizing Blends for Today's Juicers.* San Francisco: Chronicle Books, 2014.

Atlas, Nava. *Plant Power: Transform Your Kitchen, Plate, and Life with over 150 Fresh and Flavorful Vegan Recipes.* San Francisco: HarperOne, 2014.

Calabrese, Karyn. *Soak Your Nuts: Karyn's Conscious Comfort Foods—Recipes for Everyday Life.* Summertown, TN: Book Publishing Company, 2013.

Carr, Kris, with Chef Chad Sarno. *Crazy Sexy Kitchen: 150 Plant-Empowered*

Recipes to Ignite a Mouthwatering Revolution. Carlsbad, CA, and New York: Hay House, 2012.

Cornbleet, Jennifer. *Raw Food Made Easy for 1 or 2 People.* Rev. ed. Summertown, TN: Book Publishing Company, 2013.

Costigan, Fran. *Vegan Chocolate: Unapologetically Luscious and Decadent Dairy-Free Desserts.* Philadelphia: Running Press, 2013.

Cross, Joe. *The Reboot with Joe Juice Diet: Lose Weight, Get Healthy, and Feel Amazing.* Austin: Greenleaf Book Group Press, 2014.

———. *The Reboot with Joe Juice Diet Cookbook: Juice, Smoothies, and Plant-Powered Recipes Inspired by the Hit Documentary.* Austin: Greenleaf Book Group Press, 2014.

Esselstyn, Ann Crile, and Jane Esselstyn. *The Prevent and Reverse Heart Disease Cookbook: Over 125 Delicious. Life-Changing, Plant-Based Recipes.* New York: Avery Trade, 2014.

Gannon, Sharon. *Simple Recipes for Joy: More Than 200 Delicious Vegan Recipes.* New York: Avery, 2014.

Hamshaw, Gena. *Choosing Raw: Making Raw Foods Part of the Way You Eat.* Boston: DaCapo Lifelong, 2014.

Jones, Ellen Jaffe, and Alan Roettinger. *Paleo Vegan: Plant-Based Primal Recipes.* Summertown, TN: Book Publishing Company, 2014.

Kenney, Matthew. *Everyday Raw Express: Recipes in 30 Minutes or Less.* Layton, UT: Gibbs Smith, 2011.

Kirk, Mimi. *Live Raw Around the World: International Raw Food Recipes for Good Health and Timeless Beauty.* New York: Skyhorse Publishing, 2013.

Long, Linda. *Virgin Vegan: The Meatless Guide to Pleasing Your Palate.* Layton, UT: Gibbs Smith, 2013.

McCluskey, Philip. *Raw Food, Fast Food: Simple Recipes, Faster Than Takeout.* Asheville, NC: LovingRaw LLC, 2009.

Melngailis, Sarma. *Living Raw Food: Get the Glow with More Recipes from Pure Food and Wine.* New York: William Morrow Cookbooks, 2009.

Nussinow, Jill. *Nutrition CHAMPS: The Veggie Queen's Guide to Eating & Cooking for Optimum Health, Happiness, Energy, & Vitality.* Santa Rosa, CA: Vegetarian Connection Press, 2014.

Pierson, Joy, Angel Ramos, and Jorge Pineda. *Vegan Holiday Cooking from Candle Café: Celebratory Menus from New York's Premier Plant-Based Restaurants.* Berkeley, CA: Ten Speed Press, 2014.

Ranzi, Karen. *Raw Recipe Fun for Families: 115 Easy Recipes and Health Tips for Energetic Living.* Seattle: CreateSpace, 2014.

Romero, Terry Hope. *Salad Samurai: 100 Cutting-Edge, Ultra-Hearty, Easy-to-*

Make Salads You Don't Have to Be Vegan to Love. Boston: DaCapo Lifelong, 2014.

Schinner, Miyoko. *Artisan Vegan Cheese*. Summertown, TN: Book Publishing Company, 2013.

Schlimm, John. *The Cheesy Vegan: More Than 125 Plant-Based Recipes for Indulging in the World's Ultimate Comfort Food*. Boston: DaCapo Lifelong, 2013.

Soria, Cherie, and Dan Ladermann. *Raw Food for Dummies*. Hoboken, NJ: John Wiley & Sons, Inc., 2013.

Viger, Lisa. *Easy, Affordable Raw: How to Go Raw on $10 a Day*. Minneapolis: Quarry Books, 2014.

Wignall, Judita. *Raw and Simple: Eat Well and Live Radiantly with 100 Truly Quick and Easy Recipes for the Raw Food Lifestyle*. Minneapolis: Quarry Books, 2013.

Acknowledgments

......

When I read Acknowledgments from authors who thank only their editor, agent, and spouse, I'm in awe. I want to be that sophisticated and succinct, but I don't foresee it happening. Too many people help me with every book, and this one is no exception.

I will at least start with my editor, agent, and spouse—the first of those being the calm, careful, and ever so understanding Sara Carder, who believes in my work and in my message, and I'm as grateful as can be. My agent, Steve Troha, is patient, lighthearted, and really smart; I'm so lucky to be working with him. (Thanks to *Cheesy Vegan* author John Schlimm for making the introduction.) And my husband, William Melton. What can I say about a guy who met me (through a classified ad—we just missed Internet dating) and went vegetarian; who read my book, *Main Street Vegan*, and let go of the occasional delivery pizza, his last non-vegan hold-out; who moved to New York City because it was my dream; and who is in my corner nonstop? I guess I can say: I love you and appreciate you and those words aren't nearly enough.

Then come those whose contributions are a vital part of *The Good Karma Diet*:

Culinary angel Doris Fin for her mouthwatering and health-bestowing recipes;

The people whose knowledge and input helped me get things right: Neal Barnard, MD; Robert Cheeke; Nick Cooney; Terry Gips; Joel Kahn, MD; Virginia Messina, MPH, RD; Jill Nussinow, MS, RD; Karen Ranzi; Paul Shapiro; David Robinson Simon, JD; Aaron Ross; Mariann Sullivan; and the late Professor Rynn Berry, who filtered some of his vast knowledge of vegetarian history down to me, for sharing with you in chapter 21;

Demetrius J. Bagley, whose guidance of my work in the world is extraordinary;

Danielle Legg, an absolute blessing in my life, to my work, and for every nonhuman animal on this earth who's looking for a chance at a better life;

And the men and women who generously contributed their Good Karma Stories: Big Bald Mike, Patti Breitman (who was also the first person to read the manuscript and give me comments), Jenné Claiborne, Brenda Davis, RD, Chloé Jo Davis, Camille DeAngelis (who, writer to writer, helped me see what this book was meant to reveal), Dee Edwards, The Rev. Dr. Russell Elleven, Deirdre (DeDe) Gaffke, Sarah Gross, Gena Hamshaw, J. Morris Hicks, Kayle Martin, Philip McCluskey, Marissa Podany, Alan Roettinger, and Diana Tomseth. Your stories give this book its heartbeat.

Writing this book would have been much more difficult without JL Fields, VLCE, curating the MainStreetVegan.net blog; Dianne Wenz, VLCE, taking care of the Main Street Vegan Academy alumni Facebook page (and letting vegan bloggers know about *The Good Karma Diet*); and Belen Molina Prieto, VLCE, booking my speaking engagements. Nikki Keller got me away from the keyboard and into the gym, so I could write the fitness chapter with earnestness and passion. Sincere appreciation goes, as well, to Joanna Ng, my editor's assistant who approached every apparent crisis (and we did have a few!) with a lovely combination of calmness and efficiency; to publicist Angela Januzzi and publicity director Brianna Yamashita; and the many other gifted people at Tarcher/Penguin—the copy editor, cover designer, interior designer, and so many others—whose names I won't know until this manuscript becomes a book. And a perhaps unconventional but certainly heartfelt thanks to the developers of anti-social.cc, the software that excused me from e-mail and social networking in great, delicious chunks, so I could write without interruption.

Now we move to the inspirers. Any writer who doesn't partake sufficiently of the inspiration of others ends up drinking a lot. I am inspired, most of all, by my daughter, Adair Moran, a lifelong vegan, the hardest worker I know, and a young woman with what looks to me like a heap of good vegan karma. She and her husband, Nick Moran (yeah, he took her surname; cool, isn't it?), have a yard, a vegetable garden, and fruit trees *in Manhattan*. Adair acts, writes plays, works as a stunt performer, and is a New York State licensed wildlife rehabilitator and cofounder of Urban Utopia Wildlife Rehabilitation.

I am also inspired by my colleagues, women who are out to save the world and have time to support the rest of us along the way. Almost daily check-ins with Angela Kantarellis during the writing process were a godsend; Angela is a professional organizer, and just hearing her talk seemed to bring my thoughts and words into better alignment. Main Street Vegan Academy students, graduates, and faculty continue to delight me with the creative avenues they're taking to make this a saner and healthier society. The monthly support call with Fran Costigan, author of *Vegan Chocolate*, Ellen Jaffe Jones (*Eat Vegan on $4 a Day*), and Jill Nussinow, MS, RD (*Nutrition CHAMPS*) gives me the grace of community, a community that extends to include a list of other vegan authors, educators, and activists that's so long, even I will refrain from naming them all.

Index

· · · · · ·

A (adding more to your life than you subtract), 159, 164–65
Academy of Medicine, 101
Academy of Nutrition & Dietetics, 13, 107
activity resistance disorder, 186–87
additives, 224
advanced glycation end products, 155
aging process, 3, 21–22
ahimsa-based religions, 170
ALA, 34, 104
alcohol, 38–39
Altman, Nathaniel, 175
Alzheimer's, 100, 181
ama (metabolic debris), 48
Ambrosia, Tropical (recipe), 268–69
American Dietetic Association, 13, 107
American Natural Hygiene Soc., 174, 175
American Vegan Society, 174, 176
American Vegetarian Cookbook from the Fit for Life . . . (Diamond), 174
American Vegetarian Society, 171
animal agriculture
    atavistic act of, 129–31
    cultural currency, 156
    do unto others, 115–25, 157
    economics of, 138–40
    factory farming, 1–2, 6, 40, 97, 113, 115–16, 117, 131
    genetically modified organisms, 136
    Good Karma and, xii–xiii, 4, 7, 8–9, 10, 40, 90–91, 112–13
    greenhouse gases, 6, 128, 129, 161
    health problems from, 154–57
    N (never forgetting the animals), 159, 165–66
    sanctuaries, 122–23, 148
    See also Good Karma Diet; vegan; *specific animals*

Animal Liberation (Singer), 176
animal stories, 109–14
animal-testing, 160, 192, 194–95, 197
Ann Wigmore Institute, 20, 175
anthocyanins, 151
antioxidants, xiii, 18, 29, 30, 34, 100, 154, 194
Apples, Bean Dip, and Carrot Cake . . . (Dinshah and Dinshah), 64
Aries, Austin, 184
Artisan Vegan Cheese (Schinner), 9
Arundale, Rukmini Devi, 209
atavistic act of animal agriculture, 129–31
athletes, vegan, 184–85
Australia, 198
awesome ancestors, 169–77
Ayurveda, 19–20, 44, 46, 48, 79–80, 166
Ayurvedic Vegan Kitchen (Lutzker), 20

Baboumian, Patrik, 156, 184
bags (purses), vegan, 200–201
bamboo steamer, 54, 58
bananas, 62, 221
Banana Soft Serve (recipe), 267–68
Barnard, Neal, 152, 154
"barren" battery cages, 118
Bartlett, John, 202
battery cages for egg production, 118
Bauer, Ed, 184
Baur, Gene, 116
beans
    Beans 'n' Greens (recipe), 28, 37
    economics of, 138–40, 141
    Good Karma Diet, 5, 15, 16, 17, 18, 19, 21, 27, 36, 50, 78–79, 100, 105, 151, 152
    sprouting, 63–64

beans *(cont.)*
    Thai Greens and Beans (recipe), 37–38, 259–60
    Three-Bean Supreme (recipe), 250–52
    See also Good Karma Diet
beauty, fashion, shopping, 165, 191–205
Beauty and the Brunch (recipe), 227–28
Becoming Raw (Davis and Melina), 107
Becoming Vegan (Davis and Melina), 13, 107
beef cattle, 118, 119
bees and honey, 138
Beet the Competition (recipe), 226–27
before feeding yourself, nourish yourself, 87–92
Berry, Rynn, 170
Berry Brainy Smoothie (recipe), 232
Bible Christian Church, 171
Big Bald Mike's story, 187–89
Bigwood, Rob, 184
binging, 72–73
Bisci, Fred, 22
Bittman, Mark, 7
Biziou, Barbara, 192
blenders, 54–55, 244
blogs, vegan, 163
blood pressure, 66, 124, 152, 154, 156, 157, 217
blueberries, 141
"Blue Zone," Loma Linda, California, 172
body, knowing size and shape it was designed for, 71
body electric, the (spirituality), 207–12
Boldly Brilliant Borscht (recipe), 242–44
bone health, 102
Bones & All (DeAngelis), 166, 167
Book Publishing Company, 174
books, xvi, 174, 175–77, 275–79
Borscht, Boldly Brilliant (recipe), 242–44
bowls, 54
BPA caution, 28
brain fog, 101, 155
Brazier, Brendan, 184
Brazil Nut Milk (recipe), 45, 228–29
breakfasts, 33–35, 79, 80
breast cancer, 34, 97–98, 155
breathing exercises, 49
"breeders" (chicks), 117
Breitman, Patti, 90–92

British and meat-free life, 171
Broccoli Italiano (recipe), 262–63
"broilers" (chicks), 117–18
Brontë, Charlotte, 8, 177
Buckwheat Pilaf, Curried (recipe), 257–59
"Buddha bowl," 59, 62
Buddhism/Buddha, xi, 82, 83, 90, 92, 170
bulimia, 72–73
bulk shopping, 143
but everybody says something different, 147–57
"by-catch," 121

cacao, 220
Caesar Salad with Cashew Ranch (recipe), 244–46
caffeine, 35–36, 45
"cage-free" eggs, 118, 119
Calabrese, Karyn, 22
calcium, 12, 102, 157
Cameron, James, 133
Campbell, T. Colin, 16, 99, 133, 154
cancers, 18, 97–98, 100, 101, 102, 104, 123, 124, 149, 154, 155, 163, 181
Candied Carrots, 264–65
capers, 254
carbohydrates (macronutrient), 18–19, 100, 150, 151, 152, 153, 156, 157
carbon emissions, 128
cardio exercise, 47, 181–82
Carnegie Mellon University, 129
Carr, Kris, 20, 98, 211
Carter, David, 184
Cashew Ranch Dip (recipe), 244–46
cattle. *See* cows
cereal, 34–35
"chasing skinny," 70
Chavez, Cesar, 177
Cheeke, Robert, 184–85, 186, 188
cheeses, 9, 30, 172
Cheesy Caprese (recipe), 38, 249–50
Cheesy Vegan, The (Schlimm), 9
Chia Seed Pudding (recipe), 231
chickens, xiii, 1, 2, 8, 31, 40, 90, 111–12, 117–18, 120, 121, 123, 148, 188, 204
children and sprouting, 64
China, 132, 194
China Study, 16, 154

chocolate, xii, 7, 38, 114, 210
Chocolate Bliss Balls (recipe), 272–73
cholesterol, 23, 38, 124, 150, 152, 154, 156,
    217, 224
Choosing Raw (Hamshaw), 85
chopping, 224–25
Chopra, Deepak, 19
Christmas tree–looking cart and plate, 78
cinnamon, 29, 34, 96, 222
citrus juicer, 55
Claiborne, Jenné, 65–67
cleaning products, 197
Cleveland Clinic, 17, 66, 155
climate change, 94, 127–34, 138, 139, 161
Cobin, Billy James, 163
cocoa, 210
coconut, 192, 223–24
coffee grinder, 56
coffees, 35–36, 45
cold weather and eating raw, 27
collagen boosters, 194
"colony cages," 118
Community Supported Agriculture,
    142–43
Compassionate Cook (Newkirk), 174
*Compassion the Ultimate Ethic: An
    Exploration of Veganism*
    (Moran), 176
conferences, vegan, 164
Confined Animal Feeding Operation
    (CAFO), 117, 118–20, 131
connoisseur of the quotidian, 88
cookbooks, plant-powered, 174
cooking, diluting flavor, 71
Cooney, Nick, 8
Cornbleet, Jennifer, 174
Corsali, Andrea, 171
cortisol, 153
cosmetics, vegan, 192–96
Costigan, Fran, 210
Cousens, Gabriel, 20
cows, xiii, 2, 40, 97, 111–12, 113, 117, 118,
    119, 120, 121, 122, 123–24, 148,
    167, 198
Cowspiracy (documentary), 129, 131
crackers, 30
cravings, 87–88, 172
Crawford, John, 130

Crazy Sexy Cancer (Carr), 98
Crazy Sexy Diet (Carr), 20
Creamy Golden Squash Soup (recipe),
    240–42
"Creating a Charmed Life" (Moran), 219
Creating Healthy Children (Ranzi), 64
cultural currency of animals, 156
"cupcake vegans," 160
Curried Buckwheat or Quinoa Pilaf
    (recipe), 257–59
"customary agricultural practices," 116
cutting board, 54

Dagger, Bob, 215
dairy cows, 2, 40, 113, 117, 118, 120, 167
Danzig, Matt, 184
Dark Ages, 170
dark chocolate, xii, 7, 38, 210
dates, 30, 222
Davey, Marty, 161
Davis, Brenda, 11–13, 107
Davis, Chloé Jo, 203–5
Davis, Garth, 156
Davis, Glen, 185
"dead piles," 120
DeAngelis, Camille, 166–67
debt, 90
deep-breathing exercises, 49
DeGeneres, Ellen, 8
dehydrator, 30, 57
delivery food, 2
dementia, 35, 104
depression, xv, 102, 104, 188, 189, 217
desserts (recipes), 7, 36, 38, 266–73
detox program, 43–51
DHA, 101, 104–5
diabetes, 2, 6, 154, 155, 157, 181
Diamond, Harvey, 5, 176
Diamond, Marilyn, 5, 174, 176
*Dick Gregory's Natural Diet for Folks Who
    Eat* (Gregory), 173, 175
Diet for a New America (Robbins), 97, 176
Diet for a Small Planet (Lappé), 6, 139, 175
"diets" vs. Good Karma Diet, 11
dining out, 79, 213, 214–15
dinners, 37–38, 80
Dinshah, Anne and Freya, 64
Dinshah, H. Jay and Freya, 174

Diogenes, 177
dips, spreads, pâtés (recipes), 244–46, 252–55
dogs and vegetarian diets, 110–11
dollars and sense, 140–45
do unto others, 115–25, 157
doyen of the day-to-day, 88
Dr. Dean Ornish's Program for Reversing Heart Disease, 176–77
Dr. Neal Barnard's Program for Reversing Diabetes, 152
Draper, Don, 131
dry skin brushing, 49
ducks, 121, 148
Duhamel, Meagan, 185

Earhart, Amelia, 172
Earthlings (documentary), 129
Eastlund, Lois, 202
eat better/feel better, 93–98
Eating Animals (Foer), 116
eating disorders, 72–73
Eating for Life (Altman), 175
Eat to Live (Fuhrman), 17
Eat Vegan on 4 Dollars a Day (Jones, E.), 143, 174
economics, 135–45
Edison, Thomas, 172
Edwards, Dee, 39–41
E (embodying a healthy lifestyle), 159, 162–63
Ehret, Arnold, 1
electromagnetic field radiation, 46
Elleven, Russell, 123–25
Elliott, MaryJo Cooke, 184
Elvis Smoothie (recipe), 232–33
emergency kit, 7
Emerson, Ralph Waldo, 22
emotional eating, 72, 163
Engine 2 Diet, The (Esselstyn, R.), 17
English walnuts stop factor, 73
Environmental Working Group, 193
EPA, 101, 104
Esau Was onto Something Lentil Soup (recipe), 238–40
Esselstyn, Caldwell Jr., 17, 100, 133
Esselstyn, Rip, 17
essential oils, 96
"ethical vegans," 160

exercise, 47, 71, 72, 74, 163, 179–89
expense of produce, 138–39
externalized costs, 138, 139
Extraordinary Vegan (Roettinger), 24

fabrics, 201–3
Facebook, 89, 143, 163
factory farming, 1–2, 6, 40, 97, 113, 115–16, 117, 131
"far infrared" sauna, 49
Farm, The (commune in Tennessee), 174
Farm Animal Protection for the Humane Society of the United States, 119
farmers' markets, 56, 132, 136–37, 143
Farm Sanctuary: Changing Hearts and Minds... (Baur), 116
farrowing crates for pigs, 119
fashion, beauty, shopping, 165, 191–205
fast food (fruit), rethinking, 53
Fasting Can Save Your Life (Shelton), 174
Fat, Sick & Nearly Dead (documentary), 129
fats (macronutrient), 16, 18, 21, 27, 70, 72, 79, 95, 100, 149, 150, 152, 153, 154, 176, 181, 224
Fed Up (documentary), 154
feed-crops-to-humans-instead-of-livestock, 140
feng shui, 43
fermented foods, 172
festivals, vegan, 163–64
fiber (macronutrient), 51, 70, 100, 152, 154, 172
Fields, JL, 70, 252
Fife, Bruce, 48
Fin, Doris, xvi, 37–38, 45, 56, 219–25
   See also recipes
Finelli, Mary, 8
Firehouse Stew (recipe), 261–62
fishes, xiii, 8, 115–16, 119, 121, 136
Fit for Life (Diamond and Diamond), 5, 176
flesh, not eating, 8–9
Foer, Jonathan Safran, 116
foie gras trade, 198
food, health, price, justice, 135–45
food addictions, 72–73
Food and Nutrition Board of the National Academy of Science, 102

food choices, xii–xiii, 5, 12
food co-ops, 142–43
Food over Medicine (Popper), 180
Food Politics (Nestle), 144
food processor, 55
Ford, Henry, 172
Forks over Knives (documentary), 17, 129
Four Food Groups, 11
Francis (Saint), 170
Franklin, Benjamin, 111
Frazier, Matt, 185
"free-range" eggs, 118, 119
fresh juices, 29, 34, 37, 165
fruits
    desserts (recipes), 7, 36, 38, 266–73
    dried fruits, 55, 57, 104, 143, 153
    economics of, 138–40, 141
    fast food, 53
    Good Karma Diet, 2, 3, 21, 30, 34, 44,
        77, 78, 94, 95, 105, 148, 149–50,
        152, 156, 164, 194, 210
    locally grown, 137, 142
    recipes and, 220–21
    ripening, 62, 63, 137
    sugars in, 94, 151, 152
    See also Good Karma Diet
fudge, 57
Fuhrman, Joel, 17–18
full feeling, 95

Gaffke, Deirdre "DeDe," 211–12
Game Changers (documentary), 129
Gandhi, Mahatma, 172–73
Gannon, Sharon, xi–xii
gardening, 142
garlic, 28, 29, 221–22
Gaskin, Stephen, 174
gas-producing fruits, 63
"G-Bombs" (superfoods), 18
geese, 121, 148
genetically modified organisms, 136
gestation crates for pigs, 118
G (getting to know other Good Karma
    diners), 159, 163–64
Ghosts in Our Machine, The
    (documentary), 129
Gimme a V! (VEGAN acronym), 159–67
Gips, Terry, 129

GKTs. *See* Good Karma Tips
"global warming," 127
glycemic index, 19
goats, 148, 201
good cheer and a good blender
    (equipment), 53–59
Good Karma Diet, xiv–xvii, 5–13
    aging process and, 3, 21–22
    alcohol, 38–39
    breakfasts, 33–35, 79, 80
    Christmas tree-looking shopping cart
        and plate, 78
    "diets" vs., 11
    dinners, 80
    before feeding yourself, nourish
        yourself, 87–92
    food choices, xii–xiii, 5, 12
    good cheer and a good blender
        (equipment), 53–59
    Good Karma Stories, xv–xvi
    kitchen contentment, 61–67
    kitchen is closed (three meals a day vs.
        eating all day long), 74, 77–80
    legumes, 2, 3, 95, 104, 105, 142, 143, 164
    livening things up with raw foods, 22,
        25–32
    lunches, 36–37, 79–80
    making it happen, 7–10
    radiance factor, upping the, xiii–xv
    seeds, 2, 3, 18, 30, 79, 95, 105, 143, 149,
        164, 223
    skinny vs. healthy and happy, 69–76
    21 days to good health and good karma
        (detox program), 43–51
    vegetables, 2, 3, 21, 29, 78, 95, 104, 105,
        142, 164, 194, 220
    whole grains, 2, 3, 27, 45, 78, 95, 104,
        105, 142, 143, 164
    yes you can, 10–11
    See also animal agriculture; beans;
        fruits; Good Karma Tips
        (GKTs); Moran, Victoria; nuts;
        recipes; vegan; *specific stories*
Good Karma Life, 213–18
Good Karma Tips (GKTs), xv–xvi
    animal agriculture and environment, 129
    antioxidant APB, 100
    beans, 21

Good Karma Tips (GKTs) *(cont.)*
   blueberries, 141
   children and sprouting, 64
   cocoa, 210
   cold weather and raw foods, 27
   cookbooks, plant-powered, 174
   dinners, 37–38
   dogs and vegetarian diets, 110–11
   emergency kit, 7
   English walnuts stop factor, 73
   exercise, 180, 183
   fast food (fruit), rethinking, 53
   fruits, 21, 94
   full feeling, 95
   gas-producing fruits, 63
   "G-Bombs" (superfoods), 18
   genetically modified organisms, 136
   green juice daily, 28, 45
   honey and bees, 138
   hydration (water daily needs), 44
   kitchen cosmetics, 192
   language, power of, 112
   licorice tea, kicking sugar habit, 152–53
   lysine foods, 17
   mindful eating, 89
   new plant foods, getting to know, 132
   omega-3/omega-6 ratio, 105
   preparation and readiness, 10
   purging your library, 116
   red produce, collagen production, 194
   restaurants, 79, 213, 214–15
   salad, dressing up, 46
   sanctuaries, animal, 122–23, 148
   seasoned rice vinegar, 37
   sea vegetables, 19, 29, 37, 103, 172
   sense of smell, 96
   spices and antioxidants, 29
   standing vs. sitting, 162
   sunlight and vitamin D, 88, 102
   sweet potatoes, 151
   table, eating at, 82
   umami cravings, 172
   vegetables, 21
   See also Good Karma Diet
Good Morning, Good Karma (recipe), 228
Gorchynski, Stephanie, 120
government subsidies, 138, 139, 140
Graham, Douglas, 184

Graham, Sylvester, 171
granola, 30
gratitude, 88–89, 92
Great Depression, 69
Great Divide, The, 150–51
Greeña Colada (recipe), 234–35
Green Dreams (recipe), 226
greenhouse gases from animals, 6, 128,
      129, 161
green juice daily, 28, 45
Green Power Smoothie (recipe), 233–34
greens, 18, 29, 37–38, 102
green smoothies, 34, 162, 165
Greger, Michael, 6–7
Gregory, Dick, 173, 175
Gross, Sarah, 113–14
Gunn, Tim, 202

halotherapy, 49
Hamshaw, Gena, 83–85
having it your way, vegan denominations,
      15–24
health problems from meat, 154–57
      See also specific problems
"health vegans," 160
healthy and happy vs. skinny, 69–76
Healthy Eating, Healthy World (Hicks),
      128, 133
heart disease, 2, 6, 30, 100, 101, 104, 138,
      154, 155, 157, 162, 224
Heidrich, Ruth, 185
herbs and spices, 29, 142, 221–22
"he"/"she" vs. "it," 112
Hicks, Jim Morris, 128, 132–34
high-green, high-raw, high-energy eating,
      3, 33–41
Hilgart, Leanne Mai-ly, 202–3
Hinduism, xi, 170, 171
Hippocrates Health Institutes, 20, 64, 175
hiziki (hijiki) caution, 103
Holistic Heart Book, The (Kahn), 162
Holmes, Keith, 185
honey and bees, 138
horseradish, 248
hot cereal, 34–35
houseplants, 89
human contact, importance, 89
hunting, 12

Hurd, Frank and Rosalie, 174
hydration importance, 44

ice creams, 10
"If Mama ain't happy" (climate change), 6, 94, 127–34, 138, 139, 161
India, xi, 132
indulging yourself, 90
inflammation, 104, 154
Institute for Integrative Nutrition, 219
Insulin-like Growth Factor 1, 155
International Livestock Research Institute, 130
Internet retailers, 143
iodine, 103, 223
iron, 104, 156, 157
irritable bowel syndrome (IBS), xv
"I Sing the Body Electric" (Whitman), 207

Jacobson, Howard, 16, 99
Jainism, xi, 170, 171
Jefferson, Warren, 48
Jenkins, David J. A., 19
Jones, Ellen Jaffe, 19, 24, 143, 174, 185, 187, 215
Jones, James, 185
journaling experiences, 50–51
juicer, 55
juices (recipes), 225–35
Jurek, Scott, 185
just desserts, body electric, 209–11

Kafka, Franz, xiii
Kahn, Joel, 155, 162
Kaiser Permanente, 157
Kale-idoscope Salad (recipe), 246–47
karma ("action"), xi–xii, 5–6
    See also Good Karma Diet
Katcher, Joshua, 197–98, 202
Kellogg, John Harvey, 172
kelp caution, 103
Kind Diet, The (Silverstone), 19
King, Martin Luther, Jr., 173
Kirk, Mimi, 22
kitchen contentment, 61–67
kitchen cosmetics, 192
Kitchen Divided (Jones, E.), 215
kitchen economics, 141

kitchen equipment, 53–59
kitchen is closed (three meals a day vs. eating all day long), 74, 77–80
Klaper, Michael, 9
Kline, Laura, 185
knives, 54

La Fashionista Compassionista, 197, 216
language, power of, 112
Lappé, Frances Moore, 6, 139, 175
Laraque, Georges, 184
Larkins, Annette, 22
Lean Green Cream Soup (recipe), 236–37
"lean times," 69
Leaping Bunny logo, 194–95
Leaves of Grass (Whitman), 207
leftovers, 36
legumes, 2, 3, 95, 104, 105, 142, 143, 164
lemons, 29, 36, 44, 45, 55, 77, 94, 104, 224
Lentil Soup, Esau Was onto Something (recipe), 238–40
Leonardo da Vinci, 171
Le Pain Quotidien, 81
Lewis, Carl, 184
licorice tea, kicking sugar habit, 152–53
lignans, 34
"listening to your body," 87
livening things up, raw foods, 22, 25–32
Living Foods Institute in Atlanta, 98
living foods vs. raw foods, 64–65
Living Light Culinary Institute, 22
local farmers and food, 2, 19, 119, 128, 129, 136–37, 139, 142
logging experiences, 50–51
Love-Powered Diet, The (Moran), xvi
"Loving Preparation," recipes, 225
Low-Carb Fraud, The (Campbell and Jacobson), 16
lunches, 36–37, 79–80
Lutzker, Talya, 20
lycopene, 27, 194
Lyman, Howard, 130, 177
lysine, 17, 105

macrobiotics, 19
macronutrients, 100, 152–53, 161
    See also carbohydrates; fats; fiber; protein; water

macular degeneration, 101
Mad Cowboy (Lyman), 130, 177
mains (recipes), 37, 255–62
Main Street Vegan Academy, 4, 32, 163
Main Street Vegan (Moran), 116
making it happen, 7–10
Mamet, David, 81
mantras, 46, 47
manual lymphatic drainage (MLD), 50
manure lagoons, 131, 161
Marcus Aurelius, 177
Martin, Kayle, 97–98
Maslow, Abraham, 81
Masquerading Mashed "Potatoes"
    (recipe), 56, 265–66
massage, 50
May I Be Frank (documentary), 129
McCartney, Paul, 8, 179
McCartney, Stella, 202
McCluskey, Philip, 74–76
McDougall, John, 16, 17
Mead, Margaret, 213
"meat and greens" theme, 150
Meatonomics . . . (Simon), 138, 144
meditation, 46–47
Mediterranean diet, 149
Melina, Vesanto, 13, 107
melons, 221, 269
Melton, James, 2
Messina, Virginia, 105, 107, 153, 172
Metcalfe, William, 171
methane, 6, 128, 161
methionine, 155
Microgreen Garden (Braunstein), 65
microgreens, 65, 142
microwaving food, 61
Middle Ages, 170
Middle Way, 83
migraines, xv
milks, 9, 29, 45, 102, 221
Milo of Croton, 170
mindful eating, 89
mink, 198
Moore, Jeremy, 185
Moran, Victoria, xi–xvii, 211
   animal stories, 109–11
   Compassion the Ultimate Ethic: An
      Exploration of Veganism, 176

"Creating a Charmed Life," 219
   Good Karma story, 1–4, 216
   Love-Powered Diet, The, xvi
   Main Street Vegan, 116
   Main Street Vegan Academy, 4, 32, 163
   pears from Nice, France, 137
   tomatoes from Union Square farmers'
      market, 135
   See also Good Karma Diet
Morris, Jim, 184
Muesli, Super-Spa (recipe), 230
mulesing, 198, 202
muscle, plant-built, 47, 71, 72, 74, 163,
   179–89
mutilation of animals, 117–18, 120, 198
My Beef with Meat (Esselstyn, R.), 17

nasal cleansing, 48
National Health Association, 175
National Resources Defense Council, 131
Navratilova, Martina, 184
Nepal, 82–83
nerve damage, 101
Nestle, Marion, 144
Neti Pot for Better Health, The
   (Jefferson), 48
Never Diet Again (Fuhrman), 18
Never Too Late to Go Vegan
   (Breitman), 92
New Fast Food, The (Nussinow), 252
Newkirk, Ingrid, 174
new plant foods, getting to know, 132
Newton's Third Law, xii
New York City Marathon, 91
New York Times, 17, 176
Nice, France, 137
N (never forgetting the animals), 159,
   165–66
Norris, Jack, 107
North American Vegetarian Society,
   164, 176
nourishing yourself before feeding
   yourself, 87–92
numbers, letters, science, 99–107, 161
Nureyev, Rudolph, 74
Nussinow, Jill, 136–37, 252
nut mill, 56
nutritarian diet, 17–18

Nutrition and Athletic Performance
    (Graham, D.), 184
nuts
    economics of, 138–40, 141, 143
    recipes and, 220, 223
    soaking nuts, 57, 223
    vegan and, 2, 3, 30, 34, 38, 44, 50, 55,
        57, 63, 64, 65, 73, 79, 95, 105,
        148, 149, 150, 154, 164
    See also Good Karma Diet
NYC Vegetarian Food Festival, 114

Oakes, Fiona, 185–86
"oatmeal parfait," 28
obesity, 69, 71, 77–78, 136, 157
O'Hara, Scarlett (character), 87
oil pulling, 48
Oil-Pulling Therapy (Fife), 48
oils, 30, 95, 104, 136, 149, 192, 224, 260
olives, 254
omega-3s, 38, 101, 104–5, 156
omega-6s, 38, 104
One Wondrous Waldorf (recipe), 247–48
onions, 18, 221–22
Optimal Health Institutes, 20
organic foods, 139, 141, 220, 224, 254
Ornish, Dean, 100, 133, 176–77
overeating, 72–73
Owens, Montell, 185

"palate perversion," 27
Paleolithic ancestors, 161
Paleo Vegan (Jones, E. and Roettinger),
    19, 24
"Paradise Health," 1
Parks, Rosa, 177
Patel, Raj, 144
pâtés, dips, spreads (recipes), 244–46,
    252–55
Peaceable Kingdom (documentary),
    129, 204
Peaceful Palate, The (Raymond), 174
Peaches and Cream (recipe), 271–72
Pearce, Chris, 216
Perfect Health (Chopra), 19
perfectionism, pummeling, 81–85
Persistent Organic Pollutants, 155
PETA, 22, 97, 162, 176, 194

Physicians Committee for Responsible
    Medicine, 152, 164
phytochemicals, 25, 78
phyto estrogens, 149
Pie in the Sky (recipe), 270–71
pigs, xiii, 111–12, 117, 118–19, 120, 121,
    123, 148, 198, 204
Pilaf, Curried Buckwheat or Quinoa
    (recipe), 257–59
Pimentel, David, 140
plant-based, lower-carb ("Eco Atkins"),
    18–19
plant-built muscle, 47, 71, 72, 74, 163,
    179–89
PlantPure Nation (documentary), 129
Podany, Marissa, 31–32
pollution and animal agriculture,
    131, 138
Popper, Pam, 180
postpartum depression, 104
potatoes, 220
    Potatoful (recipe), 256–57
    Smashed Potatoes (recipe), 263–64
prana, 210
pregnancy, 94–95
preparation and readiness, 10
preservatives, 224
pressure cooking, 252
Presto Pesto (recipe), 254–55
Prevent and Reverse Heart Disease
    (Esselstyn, C.), 17
probiotics, 50
processed foods, 5, 16, 19, 21, 32, 43, 44,
    62, 70–71, 72, 73, 74, 104, 107, 140,
    148, 153, 154, 156, 157, 221, 224
prostate cancer, 104, 155
protein (macronutrient), 3, 12, 18–19, 34,
    58, 100, 105, 140, 150, 152, 153,
    154, 155, 156, 161, 172, 180, 183,
    186, 188
Pudding, Chia Seed (recipe), 231
pummeling perfectionism, 81–85
purging your library, 116
putting on a happy plate, 93–98
Pythagoras, 169–70

Queen of the Sun (documentary), 138
Quinoa Pilaf, Curried (recipe), 257–59

rabbits, 148
radiance factor, upping the, xiii–xv
Ranzi, Karen, 64
Raw Food, Fast Food (McCluskey), 76
raw food diet, xvi, 20–21, 37, 219, 220
    See also Good Karma Diet
Raw Food Made Easy . . . (Cornbleet), 174
Raw Food Works (Cousens), 20
Raw on $10 a Day (Viger), 143–44
Raw Recipe Fun for Families (Ranzi), 64
Raymond, Jennifer, 174
real food, more valuable than sum of its
        chemicals, 99–100, 107
recipes, xvi, 219–73
    desserts, 7, 36, 38, 266–73
    dips, spreads, and pâtés, 244–46,
        252–55
    juices, 225–35
    mains, 37, 255–62
    salads and dressings, 37, 46, 244–52
    soups, 36, 235–44
    veggie sides, 262–66
    See also Fin, Doris; Good Karma Diet
red produce, collagen production, 194
refined sugars and starches, 18, 30, 151,
        152, 153, 154, 156
Reitman, Jason, 122
resources, recipes, 225
restaurants, 79, 213, 214–15
rice and dal, 82–83
Rivera, Michelle, 111
roasted nuts and seeds, 223
Robbins, John, 97, 176
Roettinger, Alan, 19, 22–24
Roll, Rich, 185
Roman Empire, 170
Roosevelt, Eleanor, 209
Rourke, Mickey, 188
Rousey, Ronda, 185
Rozin, Yorit and Aviram, 166

Sadhana Forest, India, 166, 167
salads, 36, 45–46, 162, 213
salads and dressings (recipes), 37, 46,
        244–52
Salley, John, 184
"salt cave," 49
salts, 71, 223

sanctuaries, animal, 122–23, 148
saturated fats, 154, 156, 224
SAVE movement, 120
Save-the-Tuna Salad (recipe), 252–53
Schinner, Miyoko, 9
Schlimm, John, 9
Schweitzer, Albert, 8, 111, 177
seasonal produce, 142
sea vegetables, 19, 29, 37, 103, 172, 223
seeds, 2, 3, 18, 30, 79, 95, 105, 143,
        149, 164
selenium, 105–6
sense of smell, 96
separation, animals, 117, 120
Seventh Day Adventist Church, 171–72
Shapiro, Paul, 119, 120
Shaw, George Bernard, 172
sheep, xiii, 148, 198
"she"/"he" vs. "it," 112
Shelley, Mary, 171
Shelton, Herbert, 174
shiatsu, 50
Shields, Jake, 185
shoe business, 199–200
shopping, beauty, fashion, 165, 191–205
Shred It! (Cheeke), 184
Silverstone, Alicia, 19
Simmonds, Bill, 185
Simmons, Russell, 47
Simon, David Robinson, 138–40, 144
Simple Little Vegan Dog Book, The
        (Rivera), 111
*Simply Raw: Reversing Diabetes in 30
        Days* (documentary), 129
Simpson, Wallis, 69
Singer, Isaac Bashevis, 1–2
Singer, Peter, 176
skin (dry) brushing, 49
skinny vs. healthy and happy, 69–76
slaughtering animals, 2, 6, 115–16, 117,
        120, 121, 131, 188, 198
sleep, 46, 162, 180, 181, 209
Smashed Potatoes (recipe), 263–64
smoking, 162–63
smoothies, 28–29, 30, 34, 232–34
soaking nuts, 57, 223
Soft Serve, Banana (recipe), 267–68
Soria, Cherie, 22

soups (recipes), 36, 235–44
soy foods, 7, 9, 19, 56, 102, 104, 105, 106, 136, 149–50, 194, 221
Speciesism . . . (documentary), 129, 131
Speed Vegan (Roettinger), 23
spices and herbs, 29, 142, 221–22
spiralizer, 55
spirituality (body electric), 207–12
Spock, Benjamin, 8, 177
spreads, dips, pâtés (recipes), 244–46, 252–55
sprouted grain, 35
sprouting/sprouts, 2, 3, 17, 30, 63–64, 142
Squash Creamy Golden Soup (recipe), 240–42
Standard American Diet (SAD), 114, 156
standing vs. sitting, 162
Starch Solution, The (McDougall), 16
state of mind and desires, 93–98
steaming trivet, 54
Stew, Firehouse (recipe), 261–62
Stoudemire, Amar'e, 185
Stowe, Harriet Beecher, 8, 177
strength training, 47, 181, 182
stretching (flexibility), 47, 181, 182–83
Stuffed and Starved (Patel), 144
Success Through Stillness (Simmons), 47
sugar-sensitivity, 153
    See also refined sugars and starches
"sun-fired" bread, 35
sunlight and vitamin D, 88, 102
superfoods, 18, 142
Super-Spa Muesli (recipe), 230
sushi, 36
sweating in a "far infrared" sauna, 49
sweeteners, 30–31, 222
sweet potatoes, 38, 151

T. Colin Campbell Center for Nutrition Studies, 133
table, eating at, 82
Tapenade, Top-Drawer (recipe), 253–54
teas, 29, 35, 45, 192
Templeton, Ed, 185
Ten Talents (Hurd and Hurd), 174
Teter, Hannah, 185
Texas Beef Group, 177
Tex-Mex bar, 38

Thai Greens and Beans (recipe), 37–38, 259–60
Thai yoga massage, 50
Thoreau, Henry, 111
Three-Bean Supreme (recipe), 250–52
three meals a day vs. eating all day long, 74, 77–80
Thrive: The Vegan Nutrition Guide... (Brazier), 184
thyroid, 103
Tolstoy, Leo, 171
Tomah-To Soup, You Say (recipe), 237–38
Tomseth, Diana, 57–59
tongue cleaning, 47–48
Top-Drawer Tapenade (recipe), 253–54
Toronto Vegetarian Food Festival, 66
Transcendental Meditation, 47
transport of animals, 120–21
Tree of Life, 20
"tribe trumps everything," 163
Trimethylamine-N-oxide (TMAO), 155
Tropical Ambrosia (recipe), 268–69
Tucker, Will, 185
turkeys, xiii, 118, 121, 148
Turner, Ted, 133
21 days to good health and good karma (detox program), 43–51
28-Hour Law, 120
Twitter, 163

umami cravings, 172
undereating, 72–73
United Kingdom, 171
United States, 132, 171
Unity, 129
University of Pittsburgh, 164
University of Sydney, 130
USDA, 120

vanilla, 222
VB6 (Bittman), 7
veal calves, 117, 119
Vegan Bodybuilding and Fitness (Cheeke), 184, 186
Vegan Chocolate (Costigan), 210
Vegan for Her (Messina), 153
Vegan for Life (Norris and Messina), 107
Vegan Health and Fitness, 187

Vegan Kitchen, The (Dinshah, F.), 174
Vegan Lifestyle Coaches and Educators (VLCEs), 4, 32
vegan (no animal products of any kind, including dairy and eggs)
    awesome ancestors, 169–77
    beauty, fashion, and shopping, 165, 191–205
    body electric, the (spirituality), 207–12
    but everybody says something different, 147–57
    denominations, 15–24
    exercise, 47, 71, 72, 74, 163, 179–89
    food, health, price, justice, 135–45
    Gimme a V! (VEGAN acronym), 159–67
    Good Karma Diet, xii–xiv, xvi, 1–3, 4, 5, 6, 8–10
    high-green, high-raw, high-energy eating, 3, 33–41
    "If Mama ain't happy" (climate change), 6, 94, 127–34, 138, 139, 161
    numbers, letters, science, 99–107, 161
    plant-built muscle, 47, 71, 72, 74, 163, 179–89
    pummeling perfectionism, 81–85
    putting on a happy plate (eat better/feel better), 93–98
    See also animal agriculture; Good Karma Diet
Veganomics (Cooney), 8
Vegan Pressure Cooking (Fields), 252
Vegan Society, The, 173
vegetables, 2, 3, 21, 29, 78, 95, 104, 105, 142, 164, 194, 220
vegetarian (no meat or fish), xii, 8–9, 150
Vegetarian Nutrition Dietetic Practice Group of the American Dietetic Association, 13, 107
Vegetarian Times, 176
Veggie Fest in Hamilton, Ontario, 219
veggie sides (recipes), 262–66
Vegucated (documentary), 129
Viger, Lisa, 143–44
Vilda, 197
vitamin B$_{12}$, 9–10, 15, 101, 107, 157

vitamin C, 10, 104, 154
vitamin D, 88, 101, 102–3
vitamin D$_2$ and D$_3$, 103
vitamin K and K$_2$, 106
Vivekananda, Swami, 3
Voyevoda, Alexey, 185
V (validating your choice), 159, 160–62

Waldorf, One Wondrous (recipe), 247–48
Washington, Torre, 185
water and animal agriculture, 130, 131, 138, 139
water (macronutrient), 44, 100
Watson, Donald and Dorothy, 173
Wayne State Medical School, 155
weight loss industry rhetoric, xiv, xvii
Weissmuller, Johnny, 172
White, Ellen G., 171
Whitman, Walt, 207, 208
Whole: Rethinking . . . (Campbell and Jacobson), 99
whole-food, plant-based diet (WFPB), 16, 133
whole foods, 151, 152, 153
whole grains, 2, 3, 27, 45, 78, 95, 104, 105, 142, 143, 164
Whole Heart Solution, The (Kahn), 155
"whole-meal salad," 262
Wigmore, Ann, 175
"wild-caught" fish, 119
Williams, Serena and Venus, 185
wine, 38–39
Winfrey, Oprah, 177
winter squash, baked, 38
World Health Organization, 46, 94
world hunger, 136, 140, 144
World War II, 69, 118
wraps, 36
Wrestler, The (movie), 188

yes you can, 10–11
yoga, xi, 170, 208
You Say Tomah-To Soup (recipe), 237–38
YouTube, 22, 94, 163, 215

zinc, 106

About the Authors

. . . . . .

VICTORIA MORAN (www.MainStreetVegan.net) is an inspirational speaker and the author of twelve books, including *The Love-Powered Diet, Creating a Charmed Life,* and *Main Street Vegan,* coauthored with her daughter, Adair Moran, a lifelong vegan. Victoria hosts the weekly Main Street Vegan radio show/podcast on Unity Online Radio, and she is the founder and director of Main Street Vegan Academy, an in-person program in New York City, training people from around the world as Vegan Lifestyle Coaches and Educators (VLCEs). She lives with her husband, William Melton, and their rescue dog, Forbes, in a LEED-certified "green" condominium in Manhattan. Follow her on Facebook at Main Street Vegan, on Twitter @Victoria_Moran, and on Instagram @MainStreetVegan.

DORIS FIN (www.FeedYourBliss.com) is a Raw Food Alchemist, Certified Holistic Health Coach, and the author of *Feed Your Bliss; A Young Woman's Search for Happiness Through Taste, Touch and Travel.* While traveling the world for eight years, discovering endless flavors and colors, Doris has facilitated raw food workshops, educating and inspiring people to transform their way of eating with fun, wholesome, nutritious recipes and useful tricks for food preparation. She facilitates joyful, scrumptious, and engaging retreats in various parts of the world. Follow Doris on Facebook at Feed Your Bliss.

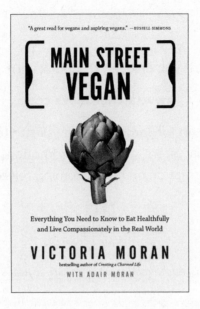

"A great read for vegans and aspiring vegans." —RUSSELL SIMMONS

MAIN STREET
VEGAN

Everything You Need to Know to Eat Healthfully
and Live Compassionately in the Real World

VICTORIA MORAN
bestselling author of *Creating a Charmed Life*
WITH ADAIR MORAN

"Finally, a book isn't preaching to the vegan choir, but to
the people in the pews—and the ones who can't fit in
those pews. This is a book for the Main Street majority
who aren't vegans. Once you read this, you'll know
it's possible to get healthy and enjoy doing it."
—Michael Moore

"Main Street Vegan...offers practical advice and inspiration
for everyone interested in going vegan, no matter
what tax bracket you're in!"
—Ellen DeGeneres

"A great read for vegans and aspiring vegans."
—Russell Simmons

If you enjoyed this book, visit

www.tarcherbooks.com

and sign up for Tarcher's e-newsletter to receive special offers, giveaway promotions, and information on hot upcoming releases.

TARCHER
PENGUIN

Great Lives Begin with Great Ideas

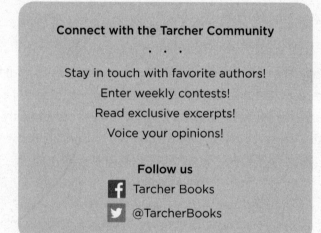

Connect with the Tarcher Community

• • •

Stay in touch with favorite authors!
Enter weekly contests!
Read exclusive excerpts!
Voice your opinions!

Follow us

Tarcher Books

@TarcherBooks

If you would like to place a bulk order of this book, call 1-800-847-5515.